Manual of Histopathological
Staining Methods

Manual of Histopathological Staining Methods

Frederick A. Putt
Department of Pathology
Yale University School of Medicine

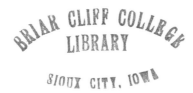

A WILEY-INTERSCIENCE PUBLICATION

JOHN WILEY & SONS , New York • London • Sydney • Toronto

Library of Congress Cataloging in Publication Data

Putt, Frederick A
    Manual of histopathological staining methods.

    Bibliography: p.
    1. Histology, Pathological–Technique. 2. Stains and staining (Microscopy)   I. Title. [DNLM: 1. Histological Technics–Laboratory manuals. 2. Stains and Staining--Laboratory manuals. QS 525 P993m 1972]

RB27.P87   6ll '.018   72-5671
ISBN 0-471-70246-3

FOREWORD

The production of a histological section requires team-
work. Usually the person who interprets the final product
also selects the tissue sample, does the initial trimming,
and starts the fixation. These are, of course, critical
steps and their importance to the usefulness of the final
product cannot be minimized. Between sending the fixed
sample to the histology laboratory and receiving the finished stained slide, however, the average pathologist or
researcher may give little thought to what is happening to
his sample. The histology technician is entrusted to handle "routinely" a thousand details of utmost importance.
Valid interpretation of the final product depends not only
on the skill of the interpreter but also on the quality of
the slide. The quality must be very good. The fairly
thin, fairly well mounted, fairly well stained, and fairly
well cleared slide is a murky forest laced with quicksand
traps and treacherous pools. The excellent preparation
may not provide all the answers, but at least it puts the
investigator on firm ground. This alone justifies the
efforts of a hard-working, skilled technician, but there
is also a bonus. A fine section is a joy to see. What
esthetic pleasure, what pure fun can come from looking
through a microscope to discover crisply sharp images in
bright clear colours!
For several years I have had the good fortune to have
slides prepared under Frederick Putt's watchful eye. Many
technicians have prepared these sections, as there have
been many students trained by this master. That the extremely high quality has been sustained by all is tes-
timony to Mr. Putt's skill as a teacher. The intricacies
of preparation of any given stain are many. The chemical
structure of the dye (when that is known) and the exact
way it functions (when that is understood) are quite
interesting and important. They are explained, discussed,
and debated in many large volumes. But the histology
technician's problem can sometimes be more immediate—he
needs to know how to make a stain "work" right now. This
manual concerns itself with how to make a stain work. The

v

small details and little tricks that make the difference
are all included. Reading from this text is the next best
thing to having a master at one's elbow.

I know from experience how useful this manual can be.
My copy of the first draft proved to be invaluable when I
was faced with setting up a laboratory in a new medical
school four years ago. Since that first draft was finished each page has been read and reread by beginners as
well as experienced technicians. This volume has thus
been subjected to extensive bench trials. I am confident
that student technicians who are just beginning to learn
their trade and experienced technicians who want to re-
fresh their memories will find this to be a manual of un-
equaled value in the laboratory. I predict that very few
copies will rest long in office or library bookcases, but
I do hope that its publication will enable me to keep a
copy near my desk. It is most aggravating to discover
that my copy has once again migrated back to the lab every
time I wish to consult it.

> Charles B. Carrington, M.D.
> Associate Professor of
> Pathology and Director of
> Autopsy Services
> Yale University School of
> Medicine

PREFACE

The histopathological staining methods presented in this manual are those with which we have had personal experience Most have been evaluated for consistency and reliability by members of the technical staff and have proved practical in routine application.

They include routine, special, and histochemical procedures as carried out in the histological laboratory in this department. Some have been modified to suit our own particular needs; others have originated from this laboratory. Classical methods which are still requested have been retained. A discussion of the all-important accessory procedures to staining, fixation, decalcification, dehydration, embedding, and sectioning is also included.

In order that a routine histological laboratory function efficiently, certain basic procedures common to various staining techniques, usually carried out in sequence, must remain fairly constant. In keeping with the needs of such a laboratory, the majority of staining methods outlined in this book can be completed during the course of a routine laboratory day. In general, the less complicated and more reproducible staining method has greater possibility of being accepted as a routine procedure. Methods that are unpredictable and that have been successful for only one or two individuals are soon rejected.

Many staining procedures share solutions in common and these could be listed together in a table. We have found it more practical, however, at the expense of repetition, to precede each method by the stated fixative of choice and the solutions necessary to complete the procedure. The reader who actually uses this manual in the laboratory will soon learn to appreciate this arrangement.

Routine, special, and histochemical methods to demonstrate related structures or tissue components are grouped together, but not in any given sequence. In some cases, more than one selection is presented in order that a choice can be made and results compared. In this manner, experience can be gained in a practical way. When checking a new or unfamiliar staining procedure, relevant control material is advisable. Because of their special applica-

tion, specific metallic and selected neuropathological
staining methods are presented separately in Chapter 12.
Many require special fixatives and are among the more
difficult techniques to master for consistent results. A
modified method to mount whole organs on paper as outlined
by Gough and Wentworth is given in Chapter 14.

Very little automation has crept into the histological
laboratory thus far. Preparing tissue for microscopic
examination is still a practical and exacting art. Many
staining methods can still be considered empirical, since
the chemical basis on which many staining reactions takes
place is not fully understood. Histochemical technique is
based on specific reactions between chemicals or dyes and
tissue components. Variation of procedure or staining
method becomes necessary at times to bring about the desired results. This will depend more on experience and
individual skill than on didactic description in a text.

Choice of tissue and proper fixative depends mostly on
the pathologist; producing acceptable histological preparations depends on the technician. Cooperation is
essential. Shoddy preparations, inadequate in detail for
diagnostic purposes, are a constant source of frustration
to the pathologist, all the more so if lectures, student
teaching, or illustrations for publication are involved.

It would be quite impossible for any one individual to
keep abreast of and evaluate current staining and related
procedures as they appear in the literature. The subject
is also too extensive for one text book to cover. For
those inclined to pursue the subject further, a list of
histological and related textbooks as well as references
to the original publications consulted in the preparation
of this manual are included.

Much of the content of this manual was formerly available
in the form of mimeographed notes. It is hoped that as-
sembling the material in book form will result in a basic
and helpful textbook for both the students and technicians
for who it is primarily intended.

In describing the various procedures and staining techniques, I have taken into consideration most of the diffi-
culties that I have personally encountered. I have tried
to present procedural details clearly and concisely in
order to avoid pitfalls. I have also benefited from
questions pertinent to a given procedure which have been
raised by members of the staff. I wish to express my
appreciation to the pathologists, technicians, and students whose stimulating questions and suggestions have
been most rewarding.

I am especially grateful to Dr. Charles Carrington for
his helpful criticism and advice, and to Dr. Klaus Bensch
and Dr. Roy Barnett for their interest and encouragement.

I am greatly indebted to Mrs. Felicia Naumann for typing
the manuscript. I also wish to thank Miss Dorothy Hyatt,
Mrs. Judy Daly, and Mrs. Gail Bliss for their technical
assistance. A textbook such as this is in great part
based on the research and experience of many authors. I
acknowledge my indebtedness to authors and publishers
who have so kindly allowed me to make use of or extract
material from their publications.

New Haven, Conn.
July, 1972   F. A. Putt

CONTENTS

TO DEMONSTRATE	METHOD
Acid-fast bacilli	Andrala's method
	Kinyoun's method
	Putt's method
	Spengler's method
	Ziehl-Neelsen method
Actinomycosis	Mallory's hematoxylin-phloxine
	Periodic acid Schiff (clubs only)
	Putt's acid fast method
Adrenals	Hematoxylin and eosin
	Masson's trichrome
	Verhoeff's elastic stain
Adrenochrome	Schmorl's Giemsa method
Amebae	Best's carmine
	Periodic acid Schiff
Amniotic fluid	Attwood's Alcian green-phloxine

TO DEMONSTRATE   METHOD

TO DEMONSTRATE	METHOD
Ferric iron	Bunting's Prussian blue reaction
	Hukill and Putt's bath-phenathroline reaction
Ferrous iron	Turnbull blue reaction
Fibrin	Heidenhain's azan carmine method
	Mallory's phosphotungstic acid hematoxylin
	Lendrum's picro-Mallory method
	Putt's fast fuchsin 6B
	Slidder's method
	Weigert's method
Fibroblasts	Heidenhain's azan carmine method
	Mallory's phosphotungstic acid hematoxylin
Fungi	Grocott's methenamine silver method
	Gridley's PAS aldehyde fuchsin method
	Giemsa method
Gastric mucin	Maxwell's Alcian green
General survey	Hematoxylin and eosin
	Hematoxylin Van Gieson
	Mallory's phosphotungstic acid hematoxylin
	Masson's trichrome
Glycogen	Bauer-Feulgen method
	Best's carmine method
Gold	Elftman's peroxide reaction
Hemofuchsin granules	Mallory's fuchsin method
Hemoglobin	Okajama's alizarine red
	Putt's benzidine-thionin
	Ralph's benzidine method
Hemosiderin iron	Mallory's hematoxylin method
Hyalin (alcoholic)	Mallory's hematoxylin-phloxine method
	Masson's trichrome stain
Hyalin droplets	Periodic acid Schiff

Contents   xix

Manual of Histopathological
Staining Methods

Chapter 1

SMEARS AND BIOPSIES

Smears are limited to tissue of a fluid of semifluid consistency such as blood or exudates. The microslides used
for this purpose should be of good quality and chemically
clean, since only tissue with a high protein content will
adhere to improperly cleaned slides. Temporary preparations, known as squashes, can be prepared from soft tissue
such as brain by gently squeezing a small sample of material between two glass microslides. These types of preparations should be fixed immediately in methyl alcohol.
Blood smears may be air-dried after fixation and stored in
a dust-free container for up to one week prior to staining, but unfixed air-dried or heat-dried specimens will
suffer loss of staining properties if saved for the same
period of time.
    Rapid and adequate preparations can be obtained by
touching the fresh-cut surface of an organ to a clean
slide, thus forming several imprints, and then fixing and
staining the adhering cells with hematoxylin and eosin,
Giemsa or Papinocolaou methods. The remaining tissue
block can then be sectioned on the cryostat or fixed and
frozen sections prepared, or processed by the paraffin
method.

CELL BLOCKS

Fluids in which the cell content is limited can be centri-
fuged. If sufficient sediment is present to form a button,
remove it carefully, place first in a Moss embedding bag
and then in tissue capsule, and process by the paraffin
method. If the material is sparse, it can be smeared on
an albuminized slide, heat-dried, and stained. (Conical-
shaped polypropylene tubes are useful to collect sediment.)

PROCEDURE

1.   Fill a clean centrifuge tube with the specimen.

*

2.   Counterbalance the centrifuge with a tube containing
      water equal in amount to the fluid being centrifuged.
3.   Centrifuge for 15 minutes at 2000 rpm. (Check amount
      collected.)
4.   Decant the supernate.
5.   Mix the sediment with 10% formalin and centrifuge
      for 15 minutes at 2000 rpm.
6.   Leave in formalin overnight.
7.   Carefully remove cell block from tube.
8.   Place in Moss embedding bag, then in tissue capsule,
      and embed in paraffin.

CRYOSTAT SECTIONING

The cryostat is essentially a refrigerated cabinet containing a rustproof microtome which permits thin sections
of unfixed tissue to be prepared for pathological diag-
nosis or histochemical procedures. The instrument should
be kept in an air-conditioned room, since excess humidity
interferes with its operation. Pearse keeps a bag of
silica jel in the cryostat and replaces it each week.
     The average sectioning temperature for routine use is
between -18° and -20°C. Tissue containing large amounts
of lipid should be sectioned at a colder setting: -23° to
-50°C. Soft cellular tissue and currettings should be
processed at a higher temperature: -10° to -20°C. A
camel's hair brush (Grumbacher, 874, No. 3), microslides,
and a spare microtome knife should be kept in the cryostat.

PROCEDURE

A piece of fresh unfixed tissue is cut no more than 2 to 5
mm in thickness with a fresh razor blade, to make the
freezing time as short as possible. It is then placed on
an object carrier, kept at room temperature, which has a
few drops of embedding compound (O.C.T.)[†] on the surface.
Multiple sections, such as currettings, can be embedded
and frozen in this material. If the carrier is at freezing
temperature, the tissue will stick and cannot be properly
oriented.
     Place the carrier on the freeze bar in the cryostat
chamber, and allow the tissue to freeze. At this point
the cover can be closed to prevent excess moisture from

*Moss embedding bags, Curtin Scientific Co. (Cat. No. 64690).
†O.C.T. embedding compound, Tissue Tec, Fisher Scientific
 Co.

entering the chamber; moisture interferes with sectioning
because it condenses and freezes on the knife edge. As
freezing progresses, the tissue turns white. To expedite
freezing, the cold quick-freeze attachment can be placed
on top of the tissue; this should be done when the tissue
is firmly attached to the carrier. When freezing is complete, a slight clockwise twist will remove the quick
freeze.

   With the microtome in the locked position, the carrier
is placed in the microtome chuck which is carefully
tightened. Set the micrometer at the desired thickness,
usually 6 microns. The microtome is unlocked, and the
tissue is ready for trimming. Be certain that the surface
of the tissue is behind the knife edge. By rocking the
hand crank on the outside of the cryostat and turning the
gross adjustment wheel when the tissue is in the uppermost position, the specimen can be gradually advanced to
the knife edge. Surface the tissue until a full section
or the desired area is reached. Debris should be carefully cleaned away with a cold camel's hair brush as it
accumulates. Once a full section has been obtained, the
knife edge should be given a final cleaning. With the
cold brush, guide the section out on the cold knife as
the block descends; the cutting action should be smooth
and continuous. We find that the brush method is more
practical than antiroll devices if the cryostat is to be
operated by various individuals.

MOUNTING

Cold Slide Method

The section is transferred from the knife to a pre-
chilled slide with a camel's hair brush and is gently
flattened. It is important that the brush be kept cold
at all times in the cryostat; otherwise the section will
adhere to the warm brush. The section is thawed by warming the area beneath the tissue with a finger; unfixed
tissue's own protein will cause it to adhere to the slide.
The thawing should be done in the cold chamber to prevent
the section from curling and accumulating excess moisture.

Warm Slide Method

As the section is cut, gently draw and flatten it on the
knife with a cold camel's hair brush. A warm slide (room
temperature) is gently lowered over the section; do not
use pressure, since the section will adhere to the slide.
Sections may also be mounted on cover glasses in a simi-

lar manner with the aid of a suction device which holds
the cover glass in position.

STORAGE

Unstained sections may be stored temporarily in a screw-
capped Coplin jar in the cryostat at -20°C until ready
for use. Generally unfixed tissue can be stored in a
sealed jar at -20°C for approximately one week; tissue
frozen in dry ice and wrapped in aluminum foil can be
stored for longer periods of time at -70°C. However, for
critical histochemical procedures tissue should be processed immediately, since stored tissue becomes dehydrated
over a period of time. Biopsy material should be fixed
immediately.

HEMATOXYLIN AND EOSIN BIOPSY STAIN (Coplin Jar Setup)

  1. Fix for 30 seconds in methyl alcohol; lipid stains
      in 10% formalin.
  2. Dip slide in Harris' hematoxylin for 30 seconds.
  3. Rinse in tap water.
  4. Dip in water containing a few drops of 28% ammonium
      hydroxide.
  5. Rinse in tap water.
  6. Counterstain in Putt's eosin solution for a few
      seconds. (p.81)
  7. Rinse in tap water.
  8. Dehydrate in two changes of absolute alcohol, 1
      minute each.
  9. Clear in xylene, two changes.
 10. Mount in Permount.

LIPID STAIN (Chiffelle and Putt method)

  1. Rinse in water to remove excess formalin.
  2. Dehydrate sections in pure propylene glycol for 3 to
      5=minutes; agitate slide gently.
  3. Transfer to flaming red in propylene glycol for
      5 minutes; see routine fat stain.
  4. Rinse sections in 85% aqueous propylene glycol for 2
      to 3 minutes.
  5. Rinse in water.
  6. Stain in Harris' hematoxylin for 2 to 3 minutes.
  7. Rinse in tap water.
  8. Blue nuclei in water containing 1 to 2 drops of 28%
      ammonium hydroxide.
  9. Rinse in water. Mount in Kaiser's glycerin jelly.

Note.   Glycerin jelly is solid at room temperature.
             Liquefy in hot water or in the incubator before
             starting procedure.

REID'S EOSIN-METHYLENE BLUE METHOD FOR BRAIN BIOPSIES

Fixation.   Formaldehyde 40% ml   15 ml
             Absolute alcohol   25 ml
             Distilled water   60 ml
             Place selected tissue in cold fixative and heat
             to boiling for 1 to 2 minutes. Squashes or smears
             of unfixed tissue may be made on clean slides
             and heat-dried.

SOLUTIONS

1.   Eosin solution.

      Eosin-Y   1 gm
      Potassium dichromate   1 gm
      Distilled water   100 ml

2.   Alcohol acetone solution.

      Acetone   50 ml
      Absolute ethyl alcohol   10 ml

3.   Methylene blue solution.

      Methylene blue   1 gm
      Potassium carbonate   1 gm
      Distilled water   300 ml
      Boil for 15 to 20 minutes. Add 3 ml of glacial acetic
      acid drop by drop and shake until the precipitate is
      dissolved. Evaporate to 100 ml and filter. The stain
      lasts for a year or more.

PROCEDURE

1.   Cut frozen sections at 20 microns into Masson's gela-
      tin water.
2.   Mount on slide and dry thoroughly on a slide warmer.
3.   Stain in eosin solution for 5 to 10 seconds.
4.   Wash carefully in distilled water.
5.   Rinse in acetone alcohol solution from dropper bottle.
6.   Wash carefully in distilled water.
7.   Stain in methylene blue solution for 10 to 30 seconds.
8.   Wash carefully in distilled water.
9.   Dehydrate and differentiate in acetone-alcohol solu-
      tion.
10.   Dehydrate in chloroform from dropper bottle.

11. Clear in xylene.
12. Mount in Permount.

Results.   Nuclei: blue. Cytoplasm: slate gray to pink.
             Collagen: pink. Blood cells: pink. Glia
             fibers: pink.

Ref.   Reid, W., Montreal Neurological Institute,
             personal communication.

HUMASON PINACYANOLE METHOD FOR FROZEN SECTIONS

SOLUTIONS

1.   Pinacyanole*   0.5 gm
     70% ethyl or methyl alcohol   100 ml

PROCEDURE

1. Mount frozen section (fresh or fixed) on subbed slide;
    drain off excess water and blot with two sheets of
    filter paper.
2. Cover section with several drops of stain: 3-5 seconds.
    (Pinacyanole,* 0.5% in either 70% methyl or ethyl
    alcohol; keep stock solution in refrigerator.)
3. Wash gently in tap water: 5-10 seconds or until free
    of excess stain (longer washing will not alter
    intensity). Blot.
4. Dehydrate in isopropyl alcohol, 2 changes: 1-2 minutes.
5. Clear in 2 changes xylene and mount.

    Because differential staining is lost in paraffin
sections, this method is recommended only for fresh or
frozen sections. In order to preserve cytoplasmic staining,
do not dehydrate the sections in ethyl or methyl alcohol;
they decolorize cytoplasmic structures, and only the
nucleus will retain appreciable amounts of stain. Steps
4 and 5 can be omitted and the sections mounted with an
aqueous mountant or glycerine.

Results.   Chromatin: well-differentiated blue to reddish
             blue. Connective tissue: pink. Elastic tissue:
             dark violet. Muscle: violet to purple. Plasma
             cells: red granuloplasm. Hemosiderin: orange.
             Hemoglobin, neutrophilic and eosinophilic
             granules: unstained. Neutral fat: colorless to
             faint bluish violet. Lipoids: bluish violet to
             purple. Amyloid: carmine red.

*Pinacyanole, Eastman Organic Chemicals, Rochester, N. Y.

faint bluish violet. Lipoids-bluish voilet to purple. Amyloid-carmine red.

Ref.   From ANIMAL TISSUE TECHNIQUES, Third Edition, by Gretchen L. Humason. W. H. Freeman and Company. Copyright © 1972.

Note.   Mounts are temporary; alcohol removes most of the stain.

HUMPHREY'S BRILLIANT CRESYL BLUE METHOD
FOR FROZEN SECTIONS

SOLUTIONS

1.   Brilliant cresyl blue   0.5 gm
      Normal saline (0.85% sodium chloride
      in distilled water   100 ml

PROCEDURE

1.   Cut formalin-fixed tissue on freezing microtome into distilled water.
2.   Mount on slide and remove excess water from edges of section with a soft towel. (Do not touch section.)
3.   Place a drop of brilliant cresyl blue on section and cover glass without rinsing.

Ref.   Humphrey, A. A., J. Lab. Clin. Med., 22 (1936-1937).

PAPANICOLAOU METHOD: EXFOLIATIVE CYTOLOGY

Fixation.   Place slides in equal parts of ether 95% alco-
            hol for 1 hour; smears should not be allowed
            to dry either before or after fixation. Smears
            to be sent through the mail should be fixed for
            1/2 hour and covered immediately with 2 to 3
            drops of glycerin. A clean slide is applied to
            serve as a cover glass; the glycerin must be re-
            moved with ether alcohol fixative before
            staining. Slides may be left for several days
            in ether alcohol in a covered Coplin jar with-
            out deterioration.
SOLUTIONS

1.   OG-6 stock solution (allow to stand for several days before use).

```
Orange-G                           10 gm
Distilled water                   100 ml
```

Working Solution
```
Orange-G 10% aqueous                5 ml
95% ethyl alcohol                  95 ml
Phosphotungstic acid            0.015 gm
```

2. EA-36 stock solution (allow to stand for several days
    before use).

```
Light green SF yellowish            2 gm
Distilled water                   100 ml

Bismarck brown Y                   10 gm
Distilled water                   100 ml
```

Alcoholic solutions

(a) 0.1% Light green SF yellowish

```
     2% aqueous light green         5 ml
     95% ethyl alcohol             95 ml
```

(b) 0.5 Bismarck brown

```
     10% aqueous Bismarck brown   5 ml
     95% ethyl alcohol            95 ml
```

(c) Eosin-Y solution

```
     Eosin-Y (water and
     alcohol soluble)            0.5 gm
     95% ethyl alcohol           100 ml
```

Working solution   (EA-36)

```
0.1 light green alcoholic
solution                          45 ml
0.5 Bismarck brown
alcoholic solution                10 ml
0.5% eosin-Y alcoholic
solution                          45 ml
Phosphotungstic acid             0.2 gm
Saturated aqueous
lithium carbonate                 1 drop
```

PROCEDURE

1. Hydrate sections through 80, 70, and 50% alcohols for a few seconds each.
2. Rinse in distilled water.
3. Stain in Harris' hematoxylin (without acetic acid) diluted to one-half with distilled water.
4. Wash very gently in running tap water for 3 to 5 minutes.
5. Differentiate in acid alcohol (0.5 hydrochloric acid in 70% alcohol).
6. Wash gently in tap water for 5 minutes.
7. Rinse for a few seconds in 50, 70, 80, and 95% alcohol.
8. Stain in OG-6 for 1 to 2 minutes.
9. Rinse in 95% alcohol, three changes for a few seconds each.
10. Stain in EA-36 or EA-50 for 2 to 3 minutes.
11. Rinse in 95% alcohol, three changes, for a few seconds.
12. Dehydrate in absolute alcohol, two changes, for one minute each.
13. Transfer to absolute alcohol xylene, equal parts, for 30 seconds.
14. Clear in xylene.
15. Mount in Permount.

Results.   Nuclei: blue. Basophil cells: blue-green or green. Acidophil cells: red to orange.

Note.   During staining do not agitate slides excessively, do not overcrowd slides in staining dish, change alcohols as they become stained, filter all stains before use and store them in brown bottles.

           EA-36, EA-50, EA-65, and OG-6 can be purchased from Ortho Pharmaceutical Corporation, Raritan, N. J.

Ref.   Emmel, V., and Cowdry, E. V., Laboratory Technique in Biology and Medicine, 4th ed., Copyright Williams and Wilkins Co., Baltimore, 1964.

Chapter 2

TISSUE FIXATION

Prompt and adequate fixation is essential to preserve
cells and tissue elements as close as possible to their
living state, including pathological changes that may
have occurred. If tissue is not fixed within a reasonable period of time, autolysis -- the self-destruction of
cells by their own enzymes -- occurs. This takes place
rapidly in enzyme producing organs, such as the pancreas,
and specialized epithelial organs, such as the kidney and
liver; it is slower in supportive tissue, such as collagen. Putrification or post mortem decomposition caused by
nonpathogenic bacteria, especially in the intestinal
tract, or by the multiplying bacteria that are present at
the time of death also cause adverse changes in tissue.
The effects of autolysis, bacterial decay, shrinkage
and drying cannot be corrected. Acceptable histoligical
preparations thus depend greatly on properly fixed tissue;
otherwise results are open to faulty interpretation.
     According to Mallory, three criteria should be con-
sidered in choosing a fixative: (1) the nature of the
tissue; (2) the nature of the pathological lesion, and
(3) the purpose for which the tissue is preserved. One
should also remember that many fixatives include mordants
to bring about specific dye reactions with tissue elements.
In some cases postmordanting can be applied prior to
staining, but the results are not so good. Other fixatives preserve certain cell or tissue products that might
be destroyed if placed in unfavorable fluids.
     Fixatives are chemical substances -- liquids, solids,
or combinations of them -- that act as coagulants or non-
coagulants on the protein of cells and tissue elements.
     Coagulating or precipitating fixatives, such as picric
acid, introduce certain artifact into tissue but leave it
in a good condition for sectioning. On the other hand,
noncoagulating fixatives, such as formalin, introduce
less artifact but tissue is left in a less satisfactory
condition. Except for formalin, acetone, and ethyl alcohol, fixatives are usually composed of three or four
chemical substances, formulated in such a manner as to

10

balance the disadvantages of one substance with the advantages of another. They also act on tissue complexes
to limit further changes when placed in such unfavorable
fluids as xylene and hot paraffin.
    Fixation is usually carried out at room temperature.
Heat can aid penetration but will also hasten post mortem
degeneration; refrigeration preserves tissue better and
does not greatly retard penetration. The practice of
keeping unfixed tissue moist with water causes the cells
to swell; this can be reduced by using physiological
saline, but leaving tissue in saline at room temperature
will not prevent autolysis. This applies especially to
surgical material, which in general receives inadequate
fixation. Excess blood and mucus on the surface of tissue
forms a film through which fixatives cannot penetrate;
these should be removed by rinsing in saline before fixation. Encapsulated material should be opened; tissue that
is prone to curl should be placed on a stiff piece of
blotting paper. Minute pieces of tissue which are apt to
be lost can be placed in Moss* embedding bags or wrapped
in lens paper. Colorless pieces should be tinted with
eosin or aqueous picric acid after fixation to make
them readily visible in paraffin.
    If it is necessary to orient tissue when embedding in
order to section a given area or to section in a certain
plane, the opposite side should be marked with a drop of
India ink; if the section is large enough a small notch
can be cut into the tissue with a razor blade after
fixation.
    The volume of fixative should be ten to twenty times
that of the tissue. Do not place tissue in an empty container without fixative; it will usually adhere to the
bottom or sides resulting in uneven penetration. For
diagnostic purposes specimens 3 to 4 mm in thickness are
desirable; if this is not practical, as in the case of
very soft tissue such as lung, after primary fixation the
tissue should be trimmed with a sharp razor blade and returned to the fixative.

SIMPLE FIXATIVES

Ethyl Alcohol

Alcohol is a reducing agent, incompatible with chromic
acid, osmium tetroxide, or potassium dichromate. Albumin
and globulin are precipitated, nucleic acid is subsequently lost. It was the fixative of choice for glycogen but

*Moss embedding bags, Curtin Scientific Co.(Cat.No.64690).

because of poor penetration, polarization occurred. Rossman's fluid is now recommended. Most lipids are dissolved;
iron, argentaffin granules, mucin, calcium, pigments, and
sodium urate are preserved. Tissue shrinks greatly,
making it difficult to stain. Hematoxylin and carmine
stains are effective. Small pieces of tissue should be
placed in cold absolute alcohol for 1 to 3 hours and kept
refrigerated during fixation. Methyl alcohol is usually
reserved for blood smears, touch preparations, and cryostat biopsy sections.

Formaldehyde

Formaldehyde is a gas, soluble to approximately 37% by
weight in water and known as 40% formalin. In routine
use a 10% solution is standard (10 ml of 40% formaldehyde to 90 ml of water). The correct term is formalin,
not formol. Over a period of time 10% formalin oxidizes
to formic acid, and the addition of calcium carbonate
(marble chips) will act as a neutralizer. Acidic formalin
reacts with blood-rich tissue to produce dark brown crystals, so-called formalin pigment. This artifact can be
prevented by the use of Lillie's buffered formalin.
Formalin is a reducing agent, incompatible with chromic
acid and osmium tetroxide, but for certain purposes can
be mixed with potassium dichromate (see Helly's fluid).
It is a slow fixative and hardens tissue fairly well but
not so much as alcohol. It causes little shrinkage, but
there may be considerable shrinkage during dehydration
and infiltration, especially if fixation is incomplete.
Formalin has little effect on neutral fats, neither pre-
serving nor destroying them. Lipids may be lost after
prolonged fixation, protein is preserved. Because of its
simplicity, formalin is generally used for routine work
and is the fluid of choice for gross tissue preservation.
It is very irritating to mucous membranes and can cause
dermatitis; hands should be protected by rubber gloves
and storage areas should be well ventilated. Hematoxylin
stains well after formalin fixation, but staining with
acid dyes is difficult.

Acetic Acid

Acetic acid is included in many fixing mixtures to coun-
teract the shrinkage effect of other chemical substances.
Like most acids, it causes tissue to swell, especially
collagen fibers, and is seldom used alone. Penetration
time is rapid, it does not fix protein, carbohydrates are
neither fixed nor destroyed, and some lipids are lost.

Many cytoplasmic granules are removed or distorted. Tissue should be washed in 70% alcohol before dehydration.

Picric Acid (Trinitrophenol)

Picric acid penetrates slowly but does not harden tissue. It causes considerable shrinkage. It appears without effect on lipids, but small fatty globules may coalesce; it does not fix carbohydrates. Proteins are precipitated forming protein picrates that enhance staining with acid dyes. There is a difference of opinion if these picric acid protein complexes are soluble in water. Tissue should be washed in 70% alcohol; part of the remaining picric acid is removed during dehydration. If basic dyes are to be used, the yellow stain can be removed before staining by including a bath of saturated lithium carbonate in 70% alcohol in the hydration series. Picric acid when dry is highly explosive and should be kept moist. It is the only chemical used as both fixative and dye.

Mercuric Chloride (Corrosive Sublimate)

This substance usually is not used alone, but is included in fixing mixtures. It may be used after initial fixation in formalin. It is a powerful precipitant of protein; has no effect on lipids but fat globules may coalesce; mucin is preserved. Penetration time is rapid for the first few millimeters, but because of its great hardening effect inner layers are underfixed and shrinkage is moderate. Tissue fixed in mercuric chloride or fixatives containing it require special treatment before staining. The crystaline mercury containing precipitate must be removed with iodine, and the iodine color removed with 5% sodium thiosulfate. Tissue fixed in mercuric chloride reacts brilliantly to most dyes.

Osmium Tetroxide (Osmic Acid)

Osmium tetroxide in a solution of water is not acid and therefore should not be termed osmic acid. It is a strong oxidizer and should not be mixed with alcohol. It is compatible with potassium dichromate and mercuric chloride. It is used to demonstrate unsaturated lipids which it blackens; other substances may also be blackened. Its penetration time is poor and uneven, leaving tissue soft; hardening occurs during dehydration leaving tissue friable and difficult to section; only small thin pieces of tissue should be processed. Staining is difficult with acid dyes, but hematoxylin and methyl green may be used. Osmium tetroxide is seldom used alone as a fixative in

histology, but is usually combined with other fixatives
such as Altmann, Marchi, and Mann's fluids. Buffered osmium tetroxide is used as a staining fixative in electron
microscopy. In solution it is very sensitive to light
and heat and should be kept in a dark, cool place in clear,
chemically clean bottles. If darkening of the solution
occurs, its potency is probably reduced. Solutions
should be handled with great care, since the vapors are
very damaging to the eyes and mucous membranes.

Chromium Trioxide (Chromic Acid)

When dissolved in distilled water, chromium trioxide
forms chromic acid--a strong oxidizing agent. It should
not be mixed with reducers such as alcohol or formalin.
It is a powerful precipitant of protein; carbohydrates
and glycogen are preserved. Penetration is very slow,
with moderate hardening and some shrinkage. Tissue must
be well washed in water after chromic acid to avoid precipitates. Tissue should not be transferred directly to
alcohol for dehydration. Cytoplasm stains well with acid
dyes.

Potassium Dichromate

This is a strong oxidizing agent and should not be mixed
with alcohol. It is not permanently stable with formalin. Unacidified dichromate is not a precipitant of protein; if acidified it acts like chromic acid and mitochondria are lost. Its hardening action is average, and
considerable shrinkage occurs during dehydration; without
additives it is a poor fixative. It enhances staining by
acid and basic dyes. Like chromic acid, dichromate-fixed
material should be washed overnight in water; precipitate
will form if tissue is transferred directly to alcohol.

FIXING MIXTURES

As pointed out previously, the action of any one simple
fixing agent is not ideal. Therefore, simple fixatives
are combined in various proportions in an effort to counterbalance undesirable effects of one substance with the
desirable effects of another.

ZENKER'S FLUID (pH 2.3)

Glacial acetic acid   5 ml
Mercuric chloride   5 gm

Potassium dichromate	2.5 gm
Distilled water	100 ml

Dissolve the mercuric chloride in one-half the distilled water with the aid of heat. Dissolve the potassium dichromate in the balance of the water. Combine the two and allow to cool. Then add the acetic acid. Zenker's dry mixture to prepare 1 or 10 liters can be obtained from Fisher Scientific Co.

Zenker's fluid is a modification of Muller's fluid to which he added acetic acid and mercuric chloride to improve the fixation of nuclei. The active fixatives in this mixture are chromic acid, acetic acid, and mercuric chloride. This fixative is a protein precipitant, cytoplasm is generally coarsely precipitated, and mitochondria and the Golgi element are destroyed. It penetrates evenly, and the cutting qualities of tissue remain good. Zenker fixed tissue must be well washed out in running water and preserved in 70% alcohol.

Tissues fixed in mercuric chloride solutions contain precipitated needle-shaped crystals thought to be mercurous chloride. These deposits must be removed before sections can be stained, which can best be accomplished prior to staining rather than on bulk tissue. After sections have been deparaffinized, they are placed in Lugol's iodine for 5 minutes, next washed in running tap water for 5 minutes, then placed in 5% sodium thiosulfate for 5 minutes, and again washed well in tap water. Almost any stain may be used after Zenker's fixation.

HELLY'S FLUID (Zenker formalin, pH 4.7)

Mercuric chloride	5 gm
Potassium dichromate	2.5 gm
Distilled water	100 ml

The basic formula for Helly's is the same as for Zenker's fluid and is prepared in the same manner. It is modified by the substitution of 5 ml of 40% formaldehyde per 100 ml of stock solution in place of acetic acid, just before use. The active fixatives in Helly's fluid are potassium dichromate, formaldehyde, and mercuric chloride. Cytoplasm and mitochrondria are well preserved. It is the fixative of choice for blood-forming organs, bone marrow, and soft tissue where decalcification is indicated. Helly fixed material is processed in the same manner as Zenker fixed tissue; as with all mercury-containing fixatives, staining is brilliant. If tissue blocks are left for an extended period of time in Zenker's or Helly's fluids, the

areas of deposit of mercuric chloride will take on a blue
coloration with hematoxylin. Metallic tissue capsules
should not be used to process tissue in mercury-containing
fixatives.

BOUIN'S FLUID (pH 1.6)

Saturated aqueous picric acid	
(1 to 1/2%)	75 ml
Formalin	25 ml
Acetic acid	5 ml

This is a good fixative for chromosomes. Cytoplasmic in-
clusions and many substances in the cell become water
soluble, and their removal results in vacuoles in the
tissue; it does not fix mitochondria and mamilliary kidney is poorly preserved. Tissue should be fixed for about
24 hours and must be washed in 70% alcohol, although
Masson prefers to soak the tissue in water. The tissue is
easily stainable, but not as brilliantly as with Helly.
If basic dyes are to be used, the yellow picric acid stain
must be removed by placing the deparaffinized sections in
a saturated solution of lithium carbonate in 70% alcohol
for a few minutes.

CARNOY'S FLUID (pH 2.7)

Glacial acetic acid	10 ml
Absolute ethyl alcohol	60 ml
Chloroform	30 ml

This is a very rapid fixative and should not be allowed
to act for longer than 1 or 2 hours. Cytoplasm and nuclei
are fixed, glycogen is precipitated and well preserved by
the alcohol, lipid and acid soluble pigments are dissolved,
myelin is lost, but Nissl granules are preserved. The
shrinkage effect is less than with plain alcohol because
of the swelling effect of the acetic acid. Tissue must
be passed directly to absolute alcohol for dehydration.
If tissue is to be embedded in celloidin, two to three
changes of absolute alcohol are necessary to remove the
chloroform. For preservation tissues should be placed in
liquid petrolatum or embedded in paraffin. Recommended
as a fixative for nucleic acids in paraffin sections.

ALCOHOLIC FORMALIN

Formaldehyde 40%	100 ml
Alcohol 95%	900 ml

Recommended to preserve glycogen. Fix under refrigeration.

ALLEN'S FLUID

Distilled water	75 ml
Formaldehyde 40%	15 ml
Glacial acetic acid	10 ml
Picric acid	1 gm
Chromic acid	1 gm
Urea	1 gm

Used as a substitute for Bouin's fluid; wash in 70% alcohol.

BAKER'S FORMALIN CALCIUM CHLORIDE

Formaldehyde 40%	100 ml
10% aqueous calcium chloride	100 ml
Distilled water	800 ml

BUNTING'S BASIC LEAD ACETATE

4% aqueous solution. Recommended for connective tissue mucins.

CAJAL'S FORMALIN-AMMONIUM-BROMIDE

Formaldehyde 40% (Merck's blue label)	15 ml
Ammonium bromide	1 gm
Distilled water	100 ml

Used to demonstrate the elements of the central nervous system by metallic methods.

FORMALIN-SALINE

Formaldehyde 40%	100 ml
Sodium chloride	8.5 ml
Distilled water	900 ml

FORMALIN-SUBLIMATE

Mercuric chloride (saturated aqueous solution)	90 ml
Formaldehyde 40%	10 ml

GENDRE'S FLUID

90% alcohol saturated with picric acid (about 9%)	85 ml
Formaldehyde 40%	10 ml
Glacial acetic acid	5 ml

Recommended to preserve glycogen; use cold; wash well with 95% alcohol.

KOLMER'S FLUID

Distilled water	87 ml
Potassium dichromate	1.8 gm
Uranyl acetate	0.75 gm
Formaldehyde 40%	3.6 ml
Glacial acetic acid	9 ml
Trichloracetic acid	4.8 gm

Recommended as a fixative for whole eyes; wash in water.

LILLIE'S ACETIC-ALCOHOL-FORMALIN

Formaldehyde 40%	10 ml
Glacial acetic acid	5 ml
Ethyl alcohol 95% to 100%	85 ml

Substitute for Carnoy's fluid.

LILLIE'S BUFFERED FORMALIN (pH 7)

Formaldehyde 40%	100 ml
Distilled water	900 ml
Acid sodium phosphate monohydrate	4 gm
Anhydrous disodium phosphate	6.5 gm

Recommended for iron and pigments, and as a general fixative to prevent the formation of formalin pigment.

LILLIE'S LEAD NITRATE FOR CONNECTIVE TISSUE MUCINS

Lead nitrate	8 gm
Formaldehyde 40%	10 ml
Distilled water	11 ml
Absolute ethyl alcohol	79 ml

Fix for 24 hours at 25 to 30°C or 0 to 5°C for 2 to 3 days. Dissolve the lead nitrate in 15 to 20 ml of dis- tilled water and add the alcohol gradually until turbidity appears; clear with a little more water and then more alco- hol, proceeding thus until a total volume of 100 ml is reached. Formalin may be included as part of the water.

MARCHI'S FLUID

Potassium dichromate	2.5 gm
Sodium sulfate	1 gm
Distilled water	100 ml

For fatty degeneration in myelin sheaths.

MULLER'S FLUID

Potassium dichromate	2.5 gm
Sodium sulfate	1 gm
Distilled water	100 ml

NEUTRAL 10% FORMALIN

Formaldehyde 40%	100 ml
Distilled water	900 ml
Calcium carbonate to excess	

ORTH'S FIXATIVE

Formaldehyde 40%	10 ml
Potassium dichromate	2.5 gm
Sodium sulfate	1 gm
Distilled water	100 ml

Good general fixative; must be made up fresh.

PETRUNKEVITCH'S FIXATIVE

60% alcohol	100 ml
Nitric acid c.p.	3 ml
Ether	5 ml
Cupric acetate c.p. crystals	2 gm
Paranitrophenol c.p. crystals	5 gm

Wash in 70% alcohol. Fixative keeps well in glass stop- pered bottles.

ROSSMAN'S FLUID

Formaldehyde 40%	10 ml
Absolute alcohol saturated with picric acid (about 9%)	90 ml

Recommended to preserve glycogen. Fix tissue in refrig‑
erator for 24 hours; wash well in 95% alcohol at room tem‑
perature.
    Calcium acetate has been suggested as a buffering agent
for formaldehyde.

Formaldehyde 40%	100 ml
Distilled water	900 ml
Calcium acetate	20 ml

    L. G. Luna and M. A. Gross [Amer. J. Med. Tech. No-
vember-December 1965] point out that an artifactual de-
position of calcium can be demonstrated in tissue by the
Von Kossa and alizarine red methods due to the use of
calcium acetate.
    D. D. Sabitini, K. G. Bensch, and R. J. Barnett [J.
Cell Biol., Vol. 17, No. 1 (1963)]introduced buffered
Glutaraldehyde* as a fixative for the electron microscope.
As a routine fixative it has proved to be superior to
formaldehyde; a 3 to 3 1/2% unbuffered solution is suitable for general purposes, the rate of penetration is
somewhat slower than formaldehyde, and prolonged immersion
in Glutaraldehyde produces a yellowing of tissue; thin
sections are therefore recommended.
    M. Yanoff, L. E. Zimmerman, and B. S. Fine [Amer. J.
Clin. Path., Vol. 44, No. 2 (1965)] recommend a 6% buffered solution of Glutaraldehyde for whole eyes.

Glutaraldehyde 25%	240 ml
Distilled water	760 ml
Monobasic sodium phosphate	1.67 gm
Dibasic sodium phosphate	16.90 gm

    Most staining procedures are improved with better
cellular preservation, the exception being the periodic
acid-Schiff reaction which is intensified. The authors
recommend treating deparaffinized sections in Lillie and
Glenner's (1957) aldehyde blocking solution for 1 hour
after exposure to periodic acid; anilin, 10 ml; glacial
acetic acid, 90 ml. Rinse in distilled water and place

*Glutaraldehyde; Union Carbide Corp., Chemical Division,
New York.

in Schiff solution. The authors also point out that acid
mucopolysaccharides demonstrated by the alcian blue and
Hale's colloidal iron reaction tend to be less intense,
and pretreatment with anilin-acetic acid solution does
not improve results.

WASHING

In most instances after fixation excess fixatives must be
removed from the tissue, since they may interfere with subsequent procedures. This is accomplished by simply washing
the tissue in running tap water. Tissue fixed in absolute
alcohol or Carnoy's fluid may be processed immediately,
as dehydration has already started. If mercuric chloride
is used in an aqueous solution, it should be washed out
in water; if in alcohol, tissue should be placed in 70%
alcohol. Most fixatives including formalin allow tissue
to be placed in 70% alcohol. The exception is tissue
fixed in mixtures containing potassium dichromate or chromic acid. These should be washed overnight, to avoid precipitates, then placed in alcohol.

STORING

After tissues have been washed, they should preferably be
dehydrated and embedded immediately. However, if this is
not convenient, tissue may be stored in 70% alcohol for a
short period of time. If prolonged, many staining reactions will be destroyed; this also applies to tissue left
for long periods of time in formalin, which oxidizes to
formic acid. Lillie's buffered formalin overcomes this
disadvantage; 10% aqueous diethylene glycol may also be
used for storage. Gross teaching specimens are best preserved in neutral 10% formalin or Brady's No. 1 fluid.
See Palkowski method.

LENDRUM'S METHOD TO SOFTEN HARD TISSUE

Place tissue after washing out the fixative in 4% aqueous
solution of phenol for 1 to 3 days, then dehydrate in the
usual manner.

Chapter 3

FROZEN-SECTION METHOD

Frozen sections permit formalin-fixed tissue to be sectioned without additional preparations; it is the method
of choice for demonstrating fatty substances. Neutral
fats are removed or dissolved in solvents used to process
paraffin or celloidin sections. Frozen sections are also
used in neurohistology to demonstrate many elements of the
central nervous system by the metallic methods of Cajal
and Hortega. Prior to the development of the cryostat,
this was the only method available for the rapid diag-
nosis of biopsy material.
     The advantage of the method of frozen sections is its
rapidity; because dehydration and especially hot paraffin
are eliminated, cells retain a lifelike appearance. The
disadvantages are that tissue may be distorted due to
freezing and cutting, sections thinner than 10 microns are
difficult to obtain, and the size of the block is limited.

CUTTING FROZEN SECTIONS

The freezing chamber on the microtome cannot be oriented;
hence tissue must be carefully trimmed, with the side to
be sectioned parallel to the opposite side and no more
that 5 mm in thickness. Before freezing, moisten the
chamber with a few drops of water, place the specimen on
the chamber, and gently hold in position with a finger.
Allow the carbon dioxide gas to escape for a few seconds
until the tissue is firmly attached, remove the finger,
and allow the gas to escape in small bursts; a continuous
stream of gas overfreezes. One can observe the progess
of freezing as the tissue turns white. Excess water on
the freezing chamber should be avoided, since it will
form compact ice and thus cause the knife to deflect.
Keep the ice level below the surface of the tissue.
     When first frozen, tissue is usually too hard to
section; allow the block to warm up to the proper cutting,
consistency. Set the micrometer at the desired thickness,
cut a few sections slowly until a full section is obtained, and then cut a number of sections in rapid succes-

sion. Cut the section by drawing the knife slowly through
the tissue. If the block is still too hard, the section
will curl or crumble; if it is too soft, the tissue will
smear on the knife or the block will separate from the
freezing chamber. Separation will also take place if
there is insufficient water between the block and freezing chamber and the tissue is overfrozen.
     As they accumulate on the knife edge, sections can be
transfered to distilled water or Masson's gelatin water
by drawing the outer edge of the little finger, slightly
moistened with water, toward the knife edge. When placed
in water they will float free. Do not allow water to
accumulate on the edge of the knife or on the surface of
the tissue; it will then freeze, resulting in streaks in
the section. If the section shreds or disintegrates
when floating in water, the block is still too hard;
sections that float rigidly are too thick. For observing
sections a black background is recommended. If sections
are to be saved for any period of time, place them in 10%
formalin. Mechanical freezing units* are available to
replace the rather bulky and unreliable carbon dioxide
tanks.

LIPID STAINS

Tissue rich in lipid is difficult to section, it usually
adheres to the warm knife as it thaws. If the knife is
chilled, reasonable sections may result. These should be
mounted on albuminized slides or on Masson's gelatin
water, and then dried and stained. If processed in the
conventional manner, most of the tissue will be lost.
This method requires increased staining time; one disadvantage is that loosely bound lipids will bleed or run
in warm mounting media.
     Usually individual frozen sections are carried
through the oil soluble dyes with the aid of a glass
"hockey stick" and finally mounted in glycerin jelly.
Small piecs of tissue, which may be lost in solution, can
be transported in a fine wire basket. A white background
facilitates the mounting of loose stained sections.

MOUNTING UNSTAINED SECTIONS (BIOPSIES)

The dish into which the sections are floated should be

*Section freeze, Lipshaw Manufacturing Co., Detroit, Mich.
 Histo freeze: Scientific Products. Tissue freeze:
 Curtin Scientific Co.

deep enough to permit a microslide to be slipped under the
the section at an angle; this is best carried out on a
black background. Choose a fairly flat section free from
folds and with a dissecting needle tease the section into
place on an albuminized slide. Gradually withdraw the
slide at an angle holding the section in place with the
needle. If the section folds, slowly lower the slide into the water holding the section in place with the needle
(the section will usually float flat) and then again
slowly withdraw the slide. Drain off excess water and
carefully pass the slide through a Bunsen flame; avoid excess heat - the slide should remain comfortable to the
touch.

Troublesome sections can be placed in 30% alcohol and
then returned to water; surface tension will cause the
section to straighten out. It is now ready to mount.

MASSON'S GELATIN WATER METHOD

One square of fine sheet gelatin* is dissolved in 100 ml
of distilled water with the aid of gentle heat; do not
allow the gelatin to burn. Filter the solution and, when
cool, add a crystal of thymol to prevent the growth of
mold. This solution is used instead of water to float
sections.

The sections are mounted as usual and then drained
and passed through a Bunsen flame until dry. Avoid excess
heat; the slide should remain comfortable to the touch.

Some workers prefer to carry unmounted sections
through the various staining solutions on a glass "hockey
stick," which should be rotated occasionally. The section
should be kept in contact with the rod, so as not to lose
it in the dye solutions. A small perforated section carrier is useful for this purpose.

MOUNTING UNFIXED FROZEN SECTIONS

Unfixed tissue is difficult to section on the freezing
microtome, especially if it is of very cellular or fatty
material; liver allows better results. Sometimes acceptable sections can be obtained with a cooled knife. As
pointed out previously, this problem has been resolved
by the cryostat method of preparing unfixed tissue, which
makes it possible to cut excellent sections of 6-micron
thickness.

*Fisher Scientific Co.

Unfixed tissue is processed in the same manner as
fixed tissue except for mounting. Because the tissue
proteins have not been altered by fixation, the tissue
can be made to adhere to the slide as follows. Drain
away the excess water while holding the slide parallel
with the working surface and then gently flood the section
with absolute alcohol from a dropper bottle, repeating
this several times. Drain off the excess fluid and allow
the section to partially dry; then place in absolute alcohol to continue fixation. Tissue prepared in this manner
cannot be used to demonstrate lipids.

GELATIN EMBEDDING

This method allows friable tissue to be sectioned on the
freezing microtome.

SOLUTION A

>   Gelatin   5 gm
>   Distilled water   100 ml
>   Phenol crystals   0.5 gm

SOLUTION B

>   Gelatin   10 gm
>   Distilled water   100 ml
>   Phenol crystals   0.5 gm

Dissolve the gelatin in water with the aid of gentle heat
(do not boil or allow to burn). Stir occasionally, allow
to cool, and add the phenol.

1.   Place blocks of tissue in solution A in 37°C oven
        and allow to infiltrate for 24 hours.
2.   Place sections in a small mold and put in solution B
        in 37°C oven for 12 hours.
3.   Transfer mold to refrigerator and allow gelatin to
        set for a maximum of 2 hours to avoid drying.
4.   Trim block and place in 10% formalin for 24 hours.

        Gelatin offers some resistance to freezing; the block
is overfrozen to ensure that the center has been frozen.
Allow the block to warm up to the proper cutting consistency and then section. When trimming block, leave as
little gelatin as possible around the tissue.
        Sections should be cut into cold water and mounted on
albuminized slides, then gently heated to coagulate the
albumin. The gelatin may be removed with warm water.
The section is now ready for staining.

Chapter 4

DECALCIFICATION

Bone and other calcified tissue require pretreatment to
remove calcium salts, which would interfere with sectioning on the microtome.

PROCEDURE

Most decalcification methods involve acid treatment and
are carried out after fixation at room temperature.
While heat accelerates the procedure, it also affects
staining because of the swelling of tissue. Vacuum and
mechanical agitators do not appear to expedite the process.
    To ensure adequate fixation, bone should be cut into
5-mm thick blocks with a fine jeweler's saw. For routine purposes, 10% formalin is recommended for compact
bone and for tissue in which iron bearing pigments are to
be preserved. Helly's fluid is preferable for the preservation of bone marrow. At times bones from young
animals or calcified tissue may be fixed and decalcified
simultaneously in Zenker's fluid. Embryonic and young
undecalcified bone can be embedded in celloidin and sectioned on the sliding microtome.
    The volume of decalcifying fluid should be about 100
times that of the tissue and should be placed in loosely
covered glass jars; metal caps should be avoided. Tissue
should not be allowed to remain in acid solutions longer
than is necessary to complete decalcification, making
allowances for the nature of the tissue--as compact or
cancellous bone or calcified tissue. An accurate check
should be kept on the progress of decalcification; if in
doubt about leaving tissue overnight, place it in 70%
alcohol and resume decalcification the following day.
    After decalcification, the block may be trimmed with
a sharp razor blade, which also serves to verify that
decalcification is complete. A crude method is to thrust
a needle into the tissue, avoiding the areas to be examined; however, spicules of bone can be missed. X-rays are
useful if available, but cannot be applied to material
fixed in mercury-containing solutions.

26

A reliable method is as follows. To 5 ml of decalcifying fluid containing specimen add 1 ml of 5% aqueous ammonium or sodium oxalate. Let stand for about 5 minutes. If the solution remains clear, decalcification is complete; if a precipitate forms, continue decalcification.

Sulkowitch's fluid may be used for the same purpose.

Malic acid	2.5 gm
Ammonium oxalate	2.5 gm
Glacial acetic acid	5 ml
Distilled water to make	50 ml

DECALCIFYING FLUIDS

The following solutions are among the many used for decalcification: 5% to 10% formic acid, 5% nitric acid, 1% to 8% hydrochloric acid, all aqueous solutions. Alcoholic solutions slow the rate of decalcification; however, if decalcifying solutions are made up in alcohol, the tissue should be washed in 70% alcohol to prevent swelling due to the combination of acid and water. For routine purposes tissue should be washed for 24 hours in running tap water. We have used the commercially prepared solution "Decal"* for a number of years with satisfactory results.

ELECTROLYTIC METHOD: IONIC BONE DECALCIFIER[†]

Decalcify in the following solution in the apparatus for 1 to 4 hours.

Formic acid 90%	100 ml
Hydrocholoric acid	80 ml
Distilled water to make	1000 ml

Wash in running tap water for 24 hours. This method depends mostly on heat causing swelling of tissue. We do not recommend this procedure.

FORMIC ACID SODIUM CITRATE

Formic acid	10 % aqueous
Sodium citrate	25% aqueous

*Decal, Scientific Products,
[†] Ionic bone decalcifier Erebach Corporation Ann Arbon, Mich.

Working solution: mix equal parts just before use; slow
acting; wash tissue well in running tap water.
Recommended for eyes.

Formic acid	5 ml
Distilled water	100 ml

Recommended for the demonstration of enzymes and the
Feulgen reaction for nuclei. Wash tissue well after decalcification.

JENKINS DECALCIFYING FIXATIVE

Concentrated hydrochloric acid	4 ml
Glacial acetic acid	4 ml
Chloroform	10 ml
Distilled water	10 ml
Absolute alcohol	73 ml

Bone about 5 mm thick is placed in a glass jar on a piece
of glass wool. Check decalcification every 5 to 6 hours;
use large amounts of solution when decalcification is
complete, wash well in several changes of absolute alcohol.

PERENYI'S DECALCIFYING FIXATIVE

Chromic acid 1% aqueous	15 ml
Nitric acid 10% aqueous	40 ml
95% alcohol	30 ml
Distilled water	15 ml

Recommended for small amounts of calcium; wash well in
70% alcohol. Keep solutions in stock, mix fresh each
time. Chemical tests to determine endpoint of decalcification do not apply to this procedure.

RAF DECALCIFYING FLUID: DOTTI, PAPARO, AND CLARKE

WIN-3000*	100 gm
10% aqueous formic acid	800 ml

Acts rapidly with good preservation of celular detail.

* WIN-3000, Special Chemicals Department, Winthrop
  Stearns, Inc., New York.

SCHMIDT'S FLUID

Formaldehyde 40%	4 ml
Distilled water	96 ml
Sodium acetate	1 gm
Disoduim versenate	10 gm

Decalcifies in 24 to 48 hours, no washing necessary, dehydrate as usual.

SCHMORL'S FLUID

Formic acid 90%	250 ml
Formaldehyde 40%	25 ml
Distilled water	225 ml

Decalcification is rapid with minimum swelling; muclei stain well.

VERSENDATE METHOD OF BIRGE AND IMHOFF

Versenate*	10 gm
Distilled water	100 ml

VON EBNER'S FLUID

Concentrated hydrochloric acid	15 ml
Sodium chloride	175 gm
Distilled water	1000 ml

Add 1 ml of hydrochloric acid per 200 ml of solution daily until decalcification is complete. Moderately rapid- about 36 hours.

Ref.   Dotti, L.B., Paparo, G.P., and Clarke, B.E. Am. J. Clin. Path 21 (1951).
Birge, E.A. and Imhoff, C.E., Am. J. Clin, Med., 22 (1952).
Jenkins, C.F., J. Path, Bact. 24 (1921).

*Disoduim dihydrogen versenate, Beersworth Chemical Co. Farmingham, Mass.

Chapter 5

PARAFFIN METHOD

DEHYDRATION

Unless otherwise indicated in keeping with the nature of the fixative, tissue blocks must be well washed in running tap water to remove excess chemicals, which cause adverse staining reactions.

Because paraffin and water are immiscible, tissue must be dehydrated before it can be infiltrated or embedded in paraffin. A number of reagents are available for this purpose. The most commonly used one is ethyl alcohol, but butyl alcohol, isopropyl alcohol, and cellosolve are also recommended. Tissue blocks are run through alcohols of increasing strength, either by hand or on an automatic tissue processor.

Paraffin is not miscible with most of the dehydrating agents except Dioxane and tetrahydrofuran, --antimedia that are compatible both with the dehydration agent and with paraffin must be inserted. Xylene, toluene, benzene, amyl acetate, chloroform, and oils such as cedarwood are a few of the reagents recommended, and are commonly termed "clearing agents" because they tend to make tissue appear translucent. The vapors of some reagents used for dehydration, such as benzene or Dioxane, are highly toxic and can also be absorbed through the skin. The area where dehydration takes place should be well ventilated.

Of the clearing agents, cedarwood oil has the least hardening effect and is useful in processing brittle tissue. Least three changes of xylene are required to remove excess oil, and then several changes of paraffin until the cedar odor is eliminated. Cedarwood oil is supplied in two forms: one for clearing tissue, the other for oil immersion. Chloroform penetrates rather slowly, and tissue does not appear as translucent as with xylene or toluene. Several changes of paraffin are necessary to remove all traces of chloroform.

Tissue blocks should never be overexposed to dehydrating or clearing agents, especially overheated paraffin.

They will become brittle and difficult to section, and staining will also be affected.

After the tissue has cleared, the antimedia must be removed and the tissue blocks infiltrated with paraffin. This is best accomplished with the aid of a vacuum oven* regulated to a few degrees above the melting point of the paraffin. Vacuum infiltration removes air from cavities within tissue and allows their refilling with paraffin. Excess vacuum should be avoided, since delicate tissue may be damaged; approximately 25 mm of mercury is sufficient. Tissue blocks run on an automatic tissue processor can be placed in vacuum for 30 minutes to complete infiltration. Small pieces of tissue, run by hand, can be infiltrated in 30 minutes in two changes of paraffin using this procedure.

Inadequately dehydrated tissue cannot be cleared or infiltrated with paraffin. When embedded, these areas will show up as opaque spots in the center of the tissue. If attempts are made to section this type of material, it will disintegrate when placed on the tissue flotation bath.

If the clearing agent is not completely removed during infiltration, it will diffuse out of the embedded tissue and soften the surrounding paraffin, causing the tissue and paraffin to separate; if sectioned, the center of the tissue will collapse.

In such cases the tissue can be salvaged; remove the excess paraffin with the aid of gentle heat, place the tissue in three to four changes of toluene for 1 hour each in the paraffin oven, and then in three or four changes of absolute alcohol at room temperature for the same period of time. Replace the tissue in toluene until clear changing when necessary, and then infiltrate and embed as usual.

Mechanical tissue-processing machines are available to carry specimens through dehydrating and clearing solutions and thermostatically controlled paraffin baths. Rotation or vertical reciprocation results in constant displacement of fluids. The duration of each step is regulated by a timing device that can be preset to suit the laboratory schedule. This procedure is usually carried out overnight. These machines form a critical part of the laboratory equipment; operating and cleaning instructions should be strictly observed, and the temperature paraffin baths checked every day.

*Thelco, Model 19, VWR Scientific.

(TECHNICON)®* DEHYDRATION SCHEDULE

SURGICAL SERVICE

4:00	6:00 p.m.	1st basket	95% alcohol + formalin
4:00	6:00 p.m.	2nd basket	95% alcohol + formalin
6:00	7:00 p.m.		Absolute alcohol
7:00	8:00 p.m.		Absolute alcohol
8:00	10:00 p.m.		Absolute alcohol
10:00	11:00 p.m.		Absolute alcohol + toluene 50/50
11:00	12:00 p.m.		Toluene
12:00	1:00 a.m.		Toluene
1:00	3:00 a.m.		Toluene
3:00	4:00 a.m.		Paraplast
4:00	6:00 a.m.		Paraplast
6:00	7:30 a.m		Paraplast

Tissues are placed for 30 minutes in vacuum oven before embedding. On weekends, the time delay clock is set to hold the Technicon until 4:00 p.m. Sunday. The first alcohol, toluene, and Paraplast should be replaced each day and the others moved up. Alcohol-formalin: 95% alcohol, 990 ml; 40% formalin, 100 ml.

AUTOPSY SERVICE

3:00	4:00 p.m.	1st basket	95% alcohol
3:00	4:00 p.m.	2nd basket	95% alcohol
4:00	5:00 p.m.		95% alcohol
5:00	8:00 p.m.		Absolute alcohol
8:00	10:00 p.m.		Absolute alcohol
10:00	11:00 p.m.		Absolute alcohol + toluene 50/50
11:00	1:00 a.m.		Toluene
1:00	3:00 a.m.		Toluene
3:00	4:00 a.m.		Toluene
4:00	6:00 a.m.		Paraplast
6:00	7:00 a.m.		Paraplast
7:00	8:30 a.m.		Paraplast

Because of their number and bulk, autopsy tissues are placed in gauze† properly identified, and bagged. This permits three to four autopsies per basket to be process-ed simultaneously. Tissues are placed for 30 minutes in vacuum oven before embedding. On weekends, the Technicon

*Technicon® Technicon Instruments Corporation. Tarrytown, N. Y. 10591.
†Folded gauze packing, 4-ply, 2-in. fold Code 8707, Johnson & Johnson. New Brunswick, N. J.

is started at 12 noon Saturday and set to change every 4
hours. Solutions should be changed as necessary.

Note. Autopsy material is fixed in Helly's fluid, washed
       and trimmed, and then sent to the laboratory in
       70% alcohol.

EMBEDDING

To facilitate the production of thin uniform tissue ribbons on the microtome, specimens must be supported by
some type of medium such as paraffin, celloidin, or
water-soluble Carbowaxes. This procedure is known as
infiltration and embedding.
      The paraffin method has the following advantages:
(1) it is rapid and simple when compared to celloidin;
(2) thin sections can be obtained; (3) ribbons of serial
sections can be cut. The disadvantages are: (1) the size
of the block is limited; (2) there is considerable shrinkage due to dehydration and infiltration, although in well
prepared tissue this artifact is uniform and constant and
in general is not detrimental for diagnostic purposes;
(3) hard tissue such as bone, skin, or muscle is cut with
difficulty.
      To improve their crystalline structure, adhesive, and
ribboning properties, making thin flat sections possible,
modern waxes used for infiltration and embedding are
modified by additives such as beeswax, bayberry wax,
asphalt, rubber, and plastic polymers.
      Commercially prepared embedding compounds are avail-
able. Tissuemat,* which contains rubber, is supplied in
a range of melting points. Paraplast,† with one melting
point, 56 to 57°C, contains plastic polymers. Both
products have good sectioning and ribboning properties
      The plastic point of paraffin determines its hardness
and is usually a few degrees below its melting point. In
the ideal situation, the melting point of paraffin would
be adapted to the temperature of the room in which
sectioning is carried out; this is not practical. Low
melting point paraffin allows thick sections of hard or
soft tissue to be cut; thinner sections can be obtained
with paraffins of a higher melting point. Paraffin with
a melting point of 56 to 58°C is suitable for routine purposes.

*Folded gauze packing, 4-ply, 2-in. fold Code 8707, Johnson
 & Johnson. New Brunswick, N. J.
†Paraplast, Tissuemat, Fisher Scientific Co.

Embedding consists of placing infiltrated tissue, properly oriented, with the surface to be sectioned face-down, into a suitable container with the aid of warm but not overheated forceps. Some tissue may have identifying marks denoting the surface to be sectioned. This usually consists of a small notch or a spot of India ink, opposite the desired surface. A slip of paper with the surgical, autopsy, or research number should accompany the specimen. It should be possible to identify tissue at any step during processing.

Paraffin used for infiltration and embedding should be filtered before use; it is advisable to keep a supply of filtered paraffin in the oven or paraffin dispenser. Embedding paraffin should be fresh and heated to about 5° above its melting point.

A variety of commercial containers and systems in which to embed tissue are available. Paper boats are the least expensive, but make the procedure time consuming. This laboratory uses the Tissue Tec* system of molds and embedding rings. The embedding ring on which the identifying number is written also acts as a block holder and is filed away with the specimen in a special cabinet; the molds are reusable. Embedding time is actually reduced, and the necessity of trimming and mounting on some type of object carrier is eliminated. When sectioning, adjustment to the microtome chuck is at a minimum. After sectioning, deblocking and tissue identification for filing purposes are no longer necessary. Tissue is instantly available for recuts without further preparation.

Tissue should be placed in paraffin while both are warm so that air will not be trapped around the tissue. (A Will Thermoplate† is useful for keeping molds and tissue warm during embedding.) This can be seen as a white halo around the tissue block after the paraffin has solidified. Usually tissues are embedded as individual blocks, but if the specimen consists of small fragments, such as currettage, they may be grouped together to form one block.

Small pieces of tissue from the same case can be embedded together so that, when they are sectioned, the knife will pass through the tissue simultaneously and not consecutively; difficulty may be encountered during sectioning if tissues represent various organs with different cutting characteristics. If it is necessary to embed thin sections on end, allow the paraffin on the bottom of the embedding boat to solidify very slightly. Tissue can then be placed in this mass and will remain upright while

*Tissue Tec, Fisher Scientific Co.
†VWR Scientific.

more paraffin is slowly added. In general, tissue should
be embedded so that when sectioned the longest plane will
be parallel with the microtome knife. Once the paraffin
has started to set, do not attempt to move the specimen.
We use a Cryo-plate* for cooling purposes; thus ice cubes,
water, and pans are eliminated, allowing tissue blocks to
be kept in an orderly fashion.

PAPER-BOAT EMBEDDING

Multiple embedding of autopsy specimens can be carried
out in large lint-free paper boats (6 x 4 x 3/4 in.),
allowing sufficient paraffin to remain on the back of the
tissue for mounting. When embedding surgical specimens,
preference is given to individual paper boats. This
eliminates the hazard of migration of small fragments,
which is possible in multiple embedding.
    Embedded blocks are left at room temperature until a
pellicle has formed on the surface of the paraffin; they
are then floated on cool water to complete solidification.
To congeal abruptly semisolid paraffin in icecold water
can be harmful to certain types of tissue. As paraffin
solidifies, its volume is reduced, which can result in
compression of soft tissue such as lung; solid tissue can
withstand the pressure better. When sectioned and floated on water, compressed tissue tends to expand to its
original size and shape; if it is confined by the paraffin
around it, pleating will result.
    Autopsy specimens embedded in large paper boats are
floated on cool water and, when sufficiently hardened,
are immersed and held down with small lead weights.
Later the paper is removed, and the block is placed in the
60°C oven, tissue side up, until pliable. This allows
individual blocks to be separated with a warm knife without splitting the paraffin.
    Blocks are trimmed of excess paraffin, leaving all
sides parallel and either square or rectangular in shape.
A small margin of paraffin is retained around the tissue.
Attach the tissue to a hardwood block by melting the
back of the paraffin with a warm spatula, letting some of
the paraffin run onto the wooden block, firmly press the
two together, and allow to solidify at room temperature.
The section should be mounted so that its longest plane
faces the knife edge. Soft wood will compress if the
microtome chuck is tightened too much, causing a fracture
between blocks, especially after exposure to ice or

*Cryo-plate, Lipshaw Manufacturing Co. Detroit, Mich.

refrigeration. Metal object carriers should be gently
heated in a Bunsen flame, then the paraffin block pressed
against it, and plunged into cold water.

CEDARWOOD OIL METHOD OF EMBEDDING

1.   95% alcohol, two changes, 2 hours.
2.   Absolute alcohol, two changes, 2 to 4 hours.
3.   Absolute alcohol and xylene, 50/50, 1 to 2 hours.
4.   Cedarwood oil (clearing type), two changes, 12 to
      24 hours.
5.   Xylene, two changes, 10 to 30 minutes.
6.   Paraplast three changes in vacuum oven, until the
      odor of cedarwood can no longer be detected.
7.   Embed in Paraplast.

Recommended for brittle tissue.

Ref. Mallory, F. B., Pathological Technique, Hafner
      Publishing Co., 1968.

METHYL BENZOATE METHOD OF DOUBLE EMBEDDING

1.   Any general fixative may be used.
2.   Wash tissue in running tap water overnight.
3.   Dehydrate in 70%, 80%, 95%, and absolute alcohol
      (time depends on size of tissue blocks).
4.   Place tissue in methyl benzoate solution for 4 hours
      or until the block sinks, then place in fresh solu-
      tion and leave overnight.

METHYL BENZOATE SOLUTION

      1 gm of celloidin in 100 ml of methly benzoate, or
      a 1% solution of celloidin in ether alcohol 50/50
      and methyl benzoate in equal parts.
5.   Place blocks in benzene to clear.
6.   Infiltrate tissue with paraffin in vacuum oven
      until no odor of benzene can be detected.
7.   Embed in paraffin.

MASSON'S AMYL ACETATE METHOD TO EMBED BRITTLE TISSUE

1.   Wash fixed tissues overnight.
2.   Place tissue in 95% alcohol for 3 hours.
3.   Place tissue in absolute alcohol for 3 hours.
4.   Absolute alchol and amyl acetate, equal parts, for
      3 hours.

5.   Amyl acetate and paraffin, equal parts in 60°C oven
     for 3 hours.
6.   Place in second change of amyl acetate and paraffin
     in oven for 3 hours.
7.   Place in fresh paraffin in the vacuum oven until the
     odor of amyl acetate cannot be detected.
8.   Embed in paraffin.

BARRON'S AMYL ACETATE PARAFFIN METHOD TO EMBED EMBRYOS

1.   Zenker's fluid.
2.   Wash in running tap water overnight.
3.   95% alcohol, 1 hour.
4.   Absolute alcohol, two changes, 2 hours.
5.   Absolute alcohol and amyl acetate 50/50, 2 hours.
6.   Amyl acetate, 24 hours.
7.   Amyl acetate and paraffin equal parts in 60°C oven,
     2 hours.
8.   Fresh paraffin, three changes.

Ref. Barron, D. H., Anat. Record, 59, 1 (1934).

DIOXANE PROCEDURE FOR PARAFFIN EMBEDDING

Diozane (1:4 diethylene dioxide) is mixable with water,
ethyl alcohol, clearing oils, and melted paraffin. It is
as inflammable as ethyl alcohol and its vapors are toxic
in concentrations of 1:1000 and should be used in a well
ventilated room. Some dioxane contains water and causes
tissue to shrink. Unless well washed, precipitated
crystals will appear in tissue fixed in Helly or Zenker's
fluids.

1.   Place fixed tissue into equal parts of dioxane and
     distilled water for 2 to 4 hours.
2.   Absolute dioxane, two changes, for 1 to 3 hours.
3.   Equal parts of dioxane and paraffin in 60°C oven for
     4 to 12 hours.
4.   Pure paraffin in 60°C oven overnight.
5.   Embed.

TETRAHYDROFURAN* (THF) FOR PARAFFIN EMBEDDING

THF is less toxic than dioxane but after prolonged exposure a slight irritation of the conjunctivae may de-

*THF, Fisher Scientific Co.

velop. It should be used in a well-ventilated room and
stock solutions should be kept tightly closed. Most
fixatives give good results. This schedule is for automatic tissue processor.

1.   10% formalin, 2 hours.
2.   10% formalin, 2 hours.
3.   THF and distilled water 50/50, 2 hours.
4.   THF (used twice), 2 hours.
5.   THF (used once), 2 hours.
6.   THF (fresh), 2 hours.
7.   THF and Paraplast 50/50, 2 hours.
8.   Paraplast, 2 hours.
9.   Paraplast, 1 hour.
10. Paraplast in vacuum oven, 30 minutes.
11. Embed.

   The solutions should be moved up every day; at step
4 replace the solution, at step 5 add fresh THF as it
evaporates, and replace it completely after 1 week.

RAPID METHOD

BRAZIL FIXATIVE

40% formaldehyde	1200 ml
Absolute alcohol	3300 ml
Picric acid	10 gm
Trichloracetic acid	22 gm

1.   Fix thin pieces of tissue in equal parts of Brazil
     and THF for 1 hour.
2.   Brazil fixative for 1 hour.
3.   THF for 30 minutes.
4.   THF for 30 minutes.
5.   THF and Paraplast 50/50 for 1 hour, in 60°C oven.
6.   Paraplast in vacuum over for 30 minutes.
7.   Embed

Ref. Haust, N. D., Lab. Investigation 7, 58-67, (1958).

CARBOWAX* METHOD: POLYETHYLENE GLYCOL, WATER-SOLUBLE WAX

1.   Any fixative may be used. Wash well in tap water.
     Helly or Zenker's fixed tissue must be washed for

*Carbowax, Carbide and Carbon Chemical Corp., New York.

at least 16 hours.   Trim blocks 3 to 4 mm in the
thickness.
2.   Carbowax solution

Carbowax 1500   1 part
Carbowax 4000   9 parts

Prepare a stock solution by placing the Carbowax in
a beaker in a 60°C oven. Do not heat over a Bunsen
burner. Keep stock solution in oven. 70% and 90%
solutions are made up with distilled water and kept
in the oven ready for use.
3.   Place sections in 70% Carbowax in the oven for 30
minutes. Occasional stirring will speed up infiltration. Fatty tissues tend to float and should be
placed in tissue capsules.
4.   Transfer to 80% Carbowax for 45 minutes and stir
occasionally.
5.   Transfer to pure Carbowax for 1 hour, stir occasionally.
6.   Embed the tissue in fresh Carbowax in a paper boat
and place in the refrigerator to harden. Do not allow water to come in contact with the block at any
time.
7.   When the wax has solidified, remove paper, trim block
with a warm knife and mount on a wooden block with
the aid of a warm spatula.

Sectioning

Sectioning is carried out in the same manner as with the
paraffin method. The brush, knife, fingers and anything
else that comes in contact with the block should be dry.
After sectioning, the blocks should be dipped in melted
Carbowax and then stored in tightly stoppered glass jars
in the refrigerator. Humidity and temperature play an important part in obtaining satisfactory ribbons.

Sections can be floated and fixed on the slide with the
following solution:

Potassium dichromate   0.2 gm
Gelatin   0.2 gm
Distilled water   1000 ml

Heat gently to dissolve. Allow mounted sections to air
dry, then place in 37°C oven for 1 hour. Store in refrigerator until ready to stain. If sections are to be used
to demonstrate lipids, all contact with alcohols and

xylene should be avoided and sections should be mounted
in glycerin jelly as routine fat stains.

<u>Ref.</u> Blank, H., J. Invest. Dermat., <u>12</u>, 95, (1949).

A METHOD TO EMBED CELL COLONIES

Individual, free-floating cell colonies, grown in liquid
agar jel, may be embedded in paraffin and sectioned as
follows.

1.   Make up a 4% solution of agar in distilled water,
      pour a thin film about 1/2-in. deep into a Petri
      dish, and allow to congeal.
2.   Cut a small block about 1/2-in. square of solid agar
      and hollow out a saucer-shaped area in the center of
      the block.
3.   Retrieve the cell colonies with a Pasteur pipette
      and collect in normal saline in a test tube. Wash
      in saline, then allow cells to settle in tube.
      Pipette off excess fluid.
4.   With the Pasteur pipette, place the cells in the
      saucer-shaped depression in the agar, add a drop of
      10% formalin, and allow cells to fix for 30 minutes.
      Withdraw the formal with a small piece of filter
      paper.
5.   Place a drop of melted agar over the cells and
      allow to solidify.
6.   Place the agar block, wrapped in lens paper in a
      tissue capsule, dehydrate, clear, and embed specimen
      side down.
7.   Cut sections of 4 to 5 microns.

PARAFFIN METHOD TO PROCESS EYES

Enucleated eyes should not be opened. Fix immediately
in Lillie's buffered formalin for 3 to 4 days in a volume of fluid at least 20 times that of the specimen.
Wash well in running tap water for 8 to 24 hours, then
place in 60% alcohol until ready for gross sectioning.

      Incise the globe with a sharp razor blade (Stadie-
Riggs*), starting several millimeters on either side of

*Stadie-Riggs, Arthur H. Thomas Co.

the optic nerve and passing through the cornea just outside the limbus. Place the center block in 80% alcohol.
At gross sectioning, if calcified material is encountered,
decalcify as follows: formic acid, 10% aqueous, sodium
citrate, 25% aqueous. Mix in equal parts just before use.
The fluid is slow acting; check progress of decalcification at regular intervals. Wash tissue well for 24 hours
in running tap water, then place in 80% alcohol or start
dehydration on automatic tissue dehydrator. Tissue,
properly identified, can be processed in embedding capsules. A separate string tag with embedding instructions
should accompany the specimen.

Technicon® Dehydration Schedule

5:00	8:00	p.m.	95%alcohol
8:00	9:00	p.m.	95% alcohol
9:00	10:00	p.m.	95% alcohol
10:00	11:00	p.m.	Absolute alcohol
11:00	12:00	p.m.	Absolute alcohol
12:00	1:00	a.m.	Absolute alcohol
1:00	2:00	a.m.	Chloroform
2:00	3:00	a.m.	Chloroform
3:00	4:00	a.m.	Chloroform
4:00	5:00	a.m.	Biloid* 56 to 58°C m.p.
5:00	6:00	a.m.	Biloid
6:00	8:00	a.m.	Biloid
8:00	8:30	a.m.	Biloid in vacuum oven

    Multiple embedding of globes in stainless steel pans[†]
is recommended. Routine material can be processed by the
Tissue Tec system as described previously. Because of the
size of the block and the nature of the tissue, globes
are best mounted on metal object carriers, to ensure
stability during sectioning.

Sectioning

1.   Section at 8 microns.
2.   Place the block in the microtome so that the sclera
      sides are parallel with the microtome knife.
3.   Trim the sections carefully until the optic nerve,
      the disc, and the pupil are exposed.
4.   Soak the surface of the tissue for several minutes
      with a piece of cotton saturated with tap water.

* Biloid embedding media, VWR Scientific.
† Stainless steel pans, Lipshaw Manufacturing Co. Detroit,
   Mich.

5.   Chill both the knife and block with ice. Before
      sectioning, the block may have be to moved back as
      the tissue swells in water. Section slowly.
6.   Two tissue flotation baths are used, the first con-
      taining distilled water at room temperature upon
      which the ribbon is floated. Individual sections are
      transfered to a second bath at 55°C, to which 3 tea-
      spoons of 5% gelatin per 1000 ml of distilled water
      have been added, and then allowed to stretch to the
      original size and shape of the block. Mount sections
      on precleaned slides.
7.   Place sections in the drying oven overnight.

Note. The gelatin water bath must be thoroughly cleaned
       after use to prevent the growth of bacteria.

Ref.   Ballou, E. F., Am. J. Med. Tech., 32, 287-291 (1966).

Chapter 6

SHARPENING AND CARE OF MICROTOME KNIVES

Once a tissue specimen has been processed up to the point of embedding, a well-sharpened microtome knife is necessary to obtain acceptable thin sections, which are essential to the proper differentiation of delicate tissue elements. This is especially important when sectioning paraffin-embedded material, in which the tissue block is thrust against the cutting edge at a 90° angle.

The sharpening of microtome knives seems to be the "bete noire" of many histological technicians, who, for one reason or another, have not learned the techniques for the proper care and use of microtome knives. Many use outside services, although even new or reconditioned knives should always be sharpened before use. If the art can be mastered, many hours of frustration at the microtome can be avoided.

Whether the fine edge of the knife is obtained by hand or on a mechanical knife sharpener, the ability to recognize a well-sharpened knife is essential. Steedman states that "90% of the successes, and 90% of the failures experienced in section cutting are due to the conditions of the microtome knife edge." Serrations or imperfections along the cutting edge must be much shallower than the thickness at which sectioning is carried out.

A microtome knife has been described as a wedge-shaped piece of steel, coming down to a fine edge -- the cutting edge; a straight line is formed by the intersection of two planes -- the cutting facets. The angle of a wedge-shaped knife is about 15°, and the cutting facets should be about 30°. Theoretically a perfect knife would be one whose extreme cutting edge has zero thickness. Such an edge is impossible because the physical properties of metals used in the manufacture of microtome knives are limited.

A knife sharpened to zero could not support the cutting edge. The extreme edge must receive support from the metal just back of the cutting edge. For this reason, older knives with larger bevels are ideal for sectioning bone and other hard objects. In time, through grinding, the knife will be reduced in size and will become useless

for sectioning, since the edge will not hold. Such knives
should be discarded.

To determine what treatment a knife should receive,
examine the entire edge under the microscope, at a
magnification of about 100. A wooden step-shaped cradle
is useful for supporting the knife while the cutting
facets are examined by reflected light. For viewing the
extreme cutting edge, the knife may be laid flat on the
microscope stage and examined by light reflected from the
microscope mirror. The extreme edge can be protected by
a piece of blotting paper placed on the stage, allowing
the edge to protrude slightly beyond the blotter. A
knife inspection microscope is now available.*

Because the steel along the cutting edge varies in
composition, it is impossible to know beforehand how a
knife will respond to sharpening. **Trial and error as well**
as cutting characteristics will determine the treatment
that each knife requires. For this reason, technicians
should have and be responsible for their own knives. To
use another's knife without permission should be regarded
as a cardinal sin.

Soft steel holds an edge poorly; very hard steel is
brittle and small pieces of the edge will sometimes break
away during sharpening, resulting in a serrated edge,
which usually cannot be repaired by stropping.

Microtome knives that today are used for paraffin
work are wedge shaped. The early hollow-ground knife is
rarely used, and the planoconcave one is reserved for
celloidin-embedded material. We have found that in general a wedge-shaped knife is suitable for all types of
material.

HAND HONING

Each knife has a back and a handle. Backs, being individually fitted to each knife, are not interchangeable and
should always be placed on the knife in the same direction
to avoid different facets on the cutting edge.

Two procedures are **available for** conditioning a knife
by hand. (1). The glass plate† method uses appropriate
abrasives such as levigated alumina for grinding, followed
by white rouge and a neutral filtered soap solution for
polishing. (2). Various types of hones or oil stones,
from coarse to fine can be used. A fine carborundum or
Norton coarse alumina will remove nicks; if the nicks are
confined to the extreme ends of the knife and do **not**

*923. Knife Inspection Microscope American Optical Corpo-
    ration, Buffalo, N.Y.
†Arthur H. Thomas Co., Philadelphia, Pa.

involve the sectioning portion the whole cutting edge need not be sacrificed, to remove them (this will only shorten the life of the knife). If the nicks are very deep, it may be necessary to return the knife to the manufacturer for reconditioning. Large nicks are usually the result of careless handling of metallic instruments near the knife edge.

The hone should be kept lubricated with a fine grade of oil such as Pike* Oil. When honing, the knife should be passed over the stone at right angles from edge to back. Sufficient pressure should be maintained with the left hand to hold the knife evenly against the stone while the right hand moves the knife. Insufficient pressure will keep the hone from taking or biting, too much pressure will produce a **feather edge**. An even number of strokes should be given to each side of the knife to avoid a burred edge; as honing progresses fresh lubricant should be added to the hone or glass plate and excessive metallic particles removed. The edge should be examined periodically to determine whether it is free of nicks.

When all large nicks have been removed, clean the knife carefully with a soft cloth moistened with xylene, rinse it in water, and then proceed to hone on a fine stone such as a Belgium blue, Arkansas white, or Norton silicone carbide, lubricated with filtered neutral soap solution, using very little pressure. Examine the edge under the microscope to determine when the coarse serrations have disappeared; as well-honed edge appears as a narrow and almost unbroken line. About 10 to 20 strokes on a fine hone will keep a nick-free knife in good condition. If this procedure is followed correctly, the knife is ready for use, and stropping will not greatly improve the edge.

STROPPING

Stropping is carried out on fine leather, which should be dressed occasionally with a high-grade oil to keep the leather supple. Strops should be kept clean and in dust-free containers when not in use. Leather strops mounted on solid blocks give the best results; a loose strop should never be used, since it will only round a well-sharpened knife.

*Pike Oil (Bear Brand), Behr-Manning Co., Division of Norton Co., Troy, N. Y.

In stopping, the knife is drawn at an angle from back
to edge with very little pressure, about four or five
strokes on each side; excessive stropping should be avoided. Before use knife should be carefully wiped clean
with a soft cloth moistened in xylene.

To test the cutting edge, set up a block of filtered
tissue-free paraffin in the microtome and cut 5-micron
ribbons; check the ribbon for striations and compression --
striations indicate a serrated or feather edge, compression, a round or dull edge. Testing the cutting edge
with a fingernail or on hairs is not advisable, as these
methods will only dull the knife.

When not in use, microtome knives should never be laid
down on the laboratory bench, since this will damage the
edge. Standing the knife on its back can be dangerous.
Instead, the knife should be carefully cleaned with a soft
cloth moistened with xylene and returned to its container.
If a knife is not to be used for a period of time, it
should be coated with light oil. We have found that well-
sharpened knives lose their keenness if left unprotected,
due to acid fumes in the laboratory.

MECHANICAL KNIFE SHARPENERS

Large institutions may find it economically feasible to
use one of the many types of mechanical sharpeners. Arthur
H. Thomas, American Optical Co., Lipshaw Manufacturing Co.,
and Curtin Scientific all supply mechanical knife sharpeners, some of which permit the technician to carry out
other duties while the knife is being processed.

A new type of microtome knife sharpener recently made
available is the Perma-Sharp. * The machine has separate
honing and stropping wheels and a fine abrasive compound
is used to dress the stropping wheels. A centrality
gage allows horizontal and verticle settings, ensuring a
reproducible cutting angle. Hand stropping is eliminated.
The complete operation takes about 5 minutes, even if the
cutting edge is badly damaged. The skill required to operate this sharpener is medium. The machine can accommodate knives up to 185 mm in length; 125-mm knives used
for the cryostat or frozen sections must be extended
slightly beyond the knife clamp to accommodate the
centrality gage. A later model will recondition knives
up to 60 cm in length. Knives should be carefully cleaned
with a soft cloth and xylene after sharpening to remove
residual stropping compounds. It has been demonstrated

*Perma-Sharp, Hacker Instruments, Inc., West Caldwell,
N. J.

by Taggart that fine amorphous particles remain on the knife edge if wiped with a dry cloth. This material has appeared in tissue sections and gives a positive Prussian blue reaction.

It would be advantageous for technicians to acquire the understanding and skill necessary to sharpen knives by hand in order to recognize a well-sharpened knife. Mechanical sharpeners are semiautomatic and are not the panacea to all knife sharpening problems; many cannot accommodate knives larger than 185 mm. Often the skill required to operate some of these machines is as great a challenge as learning to sharpen knives by hand.

Refs. Richards, O. W., The Effective Use and Proper Care of the Microtome, American Optical Co., Instruments Division, Buffalo, N. Y.
Steedman, H. F., Section Cutting in Microscopy, Blackwell Scientific Publications, Oxford, 1960.
Fanz, J. I., "An Automatic Microtome Knife Sharpener and Method for Grinding and Honing the Knife Satisfactorily," J. Lab. Clin. Med., 14 1194-1200 (1929).
Taggart, M. E., Med. Lab. Tech., 27, 36 (1970).

SECTIONING

The ability to produce and to recognize acceptable tissue sections develops only through experience. The various procedures to which tissue has been subjected up to this point play an important role in the outcome of this operation. Satisfactory sections have to be accepted or rejected by careful observation when placed on the tissue flotation bath.

For optimum staining results, especially if multiple dyes are to be applied, cells should be cut, that is, the section should not exceed the average diameter of the cell. Routine sections cut at 5 microns are satisfactory; to demonstrate specific tissue elements, however, thicker or thinner sections may be required. The following guidelines to section thickness can be used: 1 to 5 microns, thin; 5 to 10 microns medium; 10 to 50 microns, thick.

Before sectioning, all set screws holding the object carrier, knife holder, and knife must be secure to eliminate vibration; these should be hand-tightened. The microtome should not be operated with the feed mechanism extended near the limit of its excursion, or the advance mechanism will shut off. It is important to keep this in mind when serial sections are to be cut.

To produce uniform sections the microtome knife must be adjusted to the proper angle in the knife holder, with only the cutting edge coming in contact with the paraffin block. If the knife is not sufficiently inclined, the

block will drag over the cutting facet and no section will
result. This can also produce compression on the surface
of the block, which may jump forward and gouge the section. Too great an inclination will cause the paraffin
to crumble and tear the section.

In general, the tissue block should be oriented in
the microtome chuck so as to present its longest plane
to the microtome knife. It is good practice, when inserting or removing tissue blocks, to lock the microtome
drive wheel.

Before sectioning,trim excess paraffin from the face
of the block until a complete section is exposed, taking
care not to discard vital areas. Gently rock the drive
wheel on the microtome about one quarter turn, keeping
the handle in the forward position and at the same time
advancing the chuck head gradually with the feed crank
when the tissue block is in the uppermost position. In
this manner tissue may be surfaced rapidly, at the same
time eliminating the possibility of stripping the ratchet
wheel with the feed pawl.

If the bite taken is excessive, the paraffin and
tissue may crumble or they may separate from each other;
after trimming, a number of complete revolutions are made
and the first few sections are discarded. Cut a short
ribbon and examine the sections on the water bath to determine if the tissue is represented in its entirety and
whether any adjustments to the knife or microtome are
necessary.

Section thickness will vary with the nature of the
tissue, the knife edge, clearance and rake angle, room
temperature, and the rate at which sections are cut.
Cooling blocks in the refrigerator or on ice before sectioning is impractical. Ice cubes should be kept near
the microtome for any necessary cooling of the tissue
after trial sections have been made.

After the section has been surfaced, a small piece of
moist filter paper is placed over the surface of the section to prevent ice crystals from damaging the tissue.
An ice cube is now applied to the block and at times to
the knife itself, avoiding the cutting edge. This cooling
and wetting causes the tissue to swell; it is advisable to
crank back the chuck head, since the first sections will
be too thick and should be discarded.

Bloody tissue or vessels containing blood clots have
a tendency to crumble, especially if kept on ice; this
type of tissue will usually hold together if sectioned
slowly after breathing on the surface of the block. An
alternate method is to paint the surface of the block
with very thin (0.5%) celloidin dissolved in ether-
alcohol.

If the situation persists and acceptable sections are difficult to obtain, the following procedure may overcome the problem. Soak the cut surface of the paraffin block for a few hours or longer, depending on the number of sections desired, in the following solution: alcohol 70%, 90 ml; glycerin, 10 ml. The block may be left overnight in the fluid without damaging delicate tissue structures.

To section decalcified tissue, an older knife with a heavy bevel, allowing greater support behind the cutting edge set with as small a clearance angle as possible, is recommended. After surfacing bone, the first few sections should be discarded. If a tear appears in the ribbon of soft tissue and continues even after the knife is moved calcium or dirt is probably present in the paraffin; if the tear disappears, a nick probably exists at that point in the knife.

On encountering calcium when sectioning soft tissue soak the surface of the block in Decal or 2% hydrochloric acid for about 1 hour and then rinse well in water. This will allow a number of sections to be obtained without further damage to the knife edge. We use 185-mm knives for paraffin work, reserving one end for **trimming the** balance of the knife for sectioning. In this way the damage caused by any calcium or sutures **present is** limited to the trimming portion.

Sections are affected by the rate of speed at which they are cut; undue speed leads to sections of inferior **quality -- usually thicker than indicated on the micrometer. Slow sectioning is preferable to rapid sectioning,** since this increases the chance that a good uniform ribbon will result. A microtome should not be operated faster than about 100 rpm; the operation should be smooth and continuous.

If the laboratory atmosphere is dry, difficulty may be encountered due to the formation of static electricity generated by the friction of cutting. Valuable sections, especially serial sections, can be lost. This condition can be reduced by raising the humidity around the microtome or by grounding the instrument. Even better is the static eliminator, which radiates the surrounding air with alpha particles. It has been noted that rubber-soled shoes contribute to this condition. Keep the microtome and surrounding work area free of excess paraffin debris; an 1-in. paintbrush is useful.

When sectioning proceeds properly a continous straight ribbon of serial sections will result.

*Staticmaster ionizing unit, Scientific Products.

DIFFICULTIES COMMONLY ENCOUNTERED IN SECTIONING

Crooked Ribbons

Crooked ribbons are usually caused by wedge-shaped sections.

1. Correct by trimming the block so that all sides are parallel.
2. Sometimes irregularities of the knife edge causes crooked ribbons.
3. The paraffin may be softer at one end of the block than at the other. This sometimes happens to tissue that has been reembedded in paraffin of different melting point.

Sections Roll and Ribbon Fails To Form

1. The room is too cold or the paraffin is too hard. Warm the knife edge with breath, immerse in warm water, or place a lamp or Bunsen burner near the embedded object.
2. The tilt of the knife may be too great.
3. The knife may be dull - resharpen.
4. Use lower melting point paraffin.
5. Once a ribbon can be started by uncurling it with a camel's hair brush, the difficulty is frequently eliminated.

Sections Compressed, Jammed Together, or Wrinkled

1. Knife may be too dull.
2. Room may be too warm; cool blocks with ice.
3. Knife edge is not sufficiently tilted.
4. Knife edge is smeared with paraffin; clean with a soft cloth moistened with xylene.
5. The object has not been thoroughly infiltrated with paraffin.

Sections with Parallel Scratches or a Complete Fissure

1. The edge of the knife is serrated, dirty, or nicked.
2. Dirt in the paraffin.
3. Crystals from fixing fluids due to insufficient washing.
4. Tissue may contain hard substances, lime salts, silica and so on.

Sections Crumbles or Drops out of the Paraffin as Cut

1.   Alcohol not completely removed by clearing agent.
2.   Paraffin bath too hot.
3.   Too long a time in clearing fluid.
4.   Clearing agent not completely removed.
5.   Not sufficiently infiltrated with paraffin.

Sections Vary in Thickness

1.   Object clamp or knife holder or some part of the microtome is loose.
2.   Knife is not tilted sufficiently, or it is tilted too much and is polishing the section.
3.   The object may be too hard, and the edge of the knife springs.
4.   Microtome worn or not in proper adjustment.

Sections Lift from Knife on Upstroke

1.   Knife may be dull.
2.   Paraffin has accumulated on back of knife; clean with soft cloth and xylene.
3.   Room too warm; cool block with ice.

Sections Adhere to Knife

1.   Knife edge is dirty, clean with a soft cloth moistened with xylene.
2.   Increase tilt of knife.
3.   Knife edge is dull.

Scraping or Ringing Sound of Knife on Upstroke

1.   Knife tilt is slanted or too vertical.
2.   Material is too hard.
3.   A thicker wedge-shaped knife may prevent springing of the edge.

Scratching Noise during Cutting

1.   Usually caused by calcified material.
2.   Foreign material in paraffin.

Static Electricity May Cause Ribbons to Stick to Parts of Microtome

1.   Increase humidity in room.
2.   Ground microtome.
3.   Use static eliminator.

MOUNTING SECTIONS ON GLASS SLIDES

Paraffin ribbons usually have small irregularities and a
slight compression caused by wrinkles that must be extended on warm water. As the ribbon comes off the knife,
the side nearest to the cutting edge will have a shiny
surface and the uppermost side will be dull. In floating
a ribbon, the shiny surface is always laid down on the
water so that, when mounted, this surface will be in
complete contact with the microslide. If opaque areas
or bubbles remain, sections will usually float off the
slide, dyes will accumulate in the bubbles, and diffuse
out over the section when the cover glass is applied.
     There are two methods by which paraffin sections
can be mounted. In the first method a strip of ribbon is
carefully detached from the knife edge and transferred to
a tissue flotation bath* with the aid of a camel's hair
brush. (Grumbacher Series 874, No. 4.) Forceps should
not be used to remove ribbons from the knife, since this
endangers the cutting edge. The end of the ribbon held
by the brush is placed on the surface of the water at a
slight angle, the other end being held by the fingers.
It is gently lowered toward the operator, keeping a
slight but gentle tension on the ribbon, and is then
allowed to straighten out.
     The temperature of the water bath should be kept
about 10° below the melting point of the paraffin,
excessive temperature will cause the paraffin to disintegrate and the section to become unduly stretched.
This can be clearly observed in muscle tissue. Some tissue can withstand more heat than others; brain and spinal
cord require a relatively cool temperature, while other
tissue absorbs more water and becomes swollen even though
embedded in paraffin.
     The surface of the water should be kept free of
foreign material at all times. This can easily be
accomplished by drawing a wet paper towel across the surface of the water. Air bubbles trapped at the bottom or
sides of the water bath should be removed with a camel's
hair brush; these may detach themselves and settle underneath the section.
     Before mounting sections, identifying numbers must
be marked on the microslide. Slides that are frosted at
one end are convenient for this purpose; a diamond point
pencil is used on plain slides. When sectioning surgical
material, slides should be marked and tissues cut and
mounted piece by piece to aviod contamination. Autopsy

*Boekel, Arthur H. Thomas Co., Philadelphia, Pa.

material allows four to five ribbons to be sectioned from the same case and then floated and mounted on slides which can be marked in advance.

MAYER'S EGG ALBUMIN ADHESIVE

Egg whites   50 ml
Glycerin   50 ml

Beat well with an egg beater and filter through several layers of gauze in the oven. Add a crystal of thymol as a preservative. Store in refrigerator.

A small amount of albumin adhesive is spread in a thin even layer on a slide with the aid of the little finger. Excess albumin should be avoided, since it will fill in vacuoles and gather around blood vessels, absorbing dyes that cannot be removed and resulting in unsightly preparations.

At this point, examine the ribboned section critically, choose a section free from folds, bubbles, or other irregularities, and then slip a prepared slide under the section. Slowly withdraw the slide at an angle, at the same time holding the ribbon in place with a dissecting needle or camel's hair brush. The size of the section will determine how many may be mounted on the slide, allowing room for labeling. If special stains are called for and more than one slide is necessary, sections can be separated on the water bath with the aid of a dissecting needle.

Stand the slide on end in a rack and allow excess water to drain for about 5 minutes; then place in 55°C oven to complete drying and coagulate the albumin. The temperature should never be so high as to melt the paraffin.

To expedite routine hematoxylin and eosin stains, this laboratory uses metal racks* that hold 30 slides. These are loaded so that the tissue faces in the same direction, and are placed in a mechanical convection oven † regulated to 55°C. Slides may be stained in 2 hours without any further sorting; material for special stains are placed in separate racks and are usually stained in the afternoon or on the following day.

Smith A, Stain Tech., 37 (1963). has demonstrated that the temperature at which paraffin

*Staining Assembly, Arthur H. Thomas Co., Philadelphia, Pa.
†Thelco Model 18, Fisher Scientific Co.
 Ranson slide warmer, Scientific Products.

sections are dried affects subsequent staining due to
shrinkage. Sections of soft and decalcified tissue were
dried at temperatures ranging from $20^{\circ}C$ (room temperature)
to $65^{\circ}C$ and were stained with hematoxylin and eosin,
periodic acid-Schiff, and silver impregnation for reticulin and Van Gieson counterstain. Hematoxylin, eosin and
Van Gieson showed best results on soft or decalcified
tissue dried at $20^{\circ}C$.

Decalcified tissue dried at $56^{\circ}C$ showed almost complete loss of collagen by the Van Gieson counterstain;
soft tissue impregnated by silver for reticulin was best
at $56^{\circ}C$, second best at $20^{\circ}C$. Periodic acid-Schiff on
soft tissue showed an increase in intensity of staining
from 20 to $65^{\circ}C$, indicating that histochemical determin-
ations may be influenced by drying temperatures.

The second method involves the use of a Ranson slide
warmer* again regulated below the melting point of the
paraffin. A ribbon is laid on a piece of clean black
paper, and individual sections or short ribbons are
separated with a razor blade. Albuminized slides are
flooded with distilled water on the slide warmer, sections
are transfered to the slides with a moistened camel's
hair brush, and allowed to flatten. The slide is then
drained while holding the section in place with a dissecting needle. These sections are processed as by in the
previous method.

To prepare slides for 35-mm projection, we have for a
number of years mounted paraffin sections on 50 x 50 mm
(2 x 2 in.) thin Kodak slide cover glasses, using a second cover glass as the cover slip. Identification should
be written in opposite the slide on which tissue is
mounted; markings become illegible in mounting media.

These are processed and stained as usual, after mounting
in Permount (which, because of its high melting point
150°, can withstand projection heat). Slides are left
in the $50^{\circ}C$ oven overnight to dry and then are bound
with binding tape or inserted in aluminum slide binders.[†]
A staining rack supplied by Lipshaw Manufacturing Co.[‡]
(No. 114) is ideal to carry this type of slide through
the various solutions.

SERIAL SECTIONS

When complete serial sections are necessary, ribbons that
can be handled conveniently of 10 to 20 sections depending

*Ranson Slide Warmer Scientific Products
†EMDE Products Inc., Los Angeles, Calif.
‡Lipshaw Manufacturing Co., Detroit, Mich.

on the size of the block are cut and laid in numerical order in a dust-free container. Cut a small triangular wedge from the four corners of the block before sectioning; this will separate the individual sections by a V-shaped notch. The top of the first ribbon is labeled 1, the next 11 or 21, and so on. Each layer of ribbons may be separated by a thin sheet of black paper; in this manner serial sections can be sectioned rapidly and stored in the refrigerator until ready for mounting.

When removing ribbon from the knife, separate the ribbon at a distance from the knife edge, leaving a few segments attached; in this way loss of sections between ribbons is prevented. To avoid disaster this procedure should be carried out in a draft-free room behind locked doors.

With the aid of a camel's hair brush, individual ribbons are floated on the water bath and the sections separated with a sharp dissecting needle along the line of the V-shaped notch; to prevent damage, forceps should not be used to lift sections. The sections should be mounted in the numerical order indicated on the slide and all in the same direction so that during microscopical examination it will not be necessary to continually rotate the slide in order to view the same area. If multiple small sections are to be mounted on the same slide, the slide warmer method is preferred.

Partial serial sections can be obtained by discarding either 5 or 10 sections between the sections saved. It is preferable to mount the sections immediately on numbered slides.

An alternate method of affixing sections to micro-slides is Masson's* gelatin water. In this procedure the finest French sheet gelatin must be used (Coignet, Pere & Fils & Cie, Silver Label†). One square of gelatin is cut into small pieces with a pair of scissors, is allowed to stand in 100 ml of distilled water for 1/2 hour, and then is gently heated, stirring constantly to prevent the gelatin from burning; filter and add a crystal of thymol when cool to prevent the growth of mold.

Ref. Dempster, W. T., "Paraffin compression due to the
      rotary Microtome," Stain Tech., 18, 13-24 (1924).

*P. Masson, Am. J. Path., 4 181, (1928).
†Silver label sheet gelatin, Fisher Scientific Co.

Sections are mounted using the slide warmer method; a dropper bottle may be used to flood the slides with gelatin water. After draining, slides are placed in a 37°C incubator with an open Stender dish containing 40% formaldehyde; 2 hours is sufficient for routine stains. This procedure is extremely useful for metallic impregnations, brain, and bone sections which should be left overnight in the incubator. Caution must be exercised when opening the oven because of the formalin fumes.

CARE OF THE MICROTOME

Before operating the microtome all sliding surfaces should be examined and if necessary oiled with Pike oil,* especially the celloidin microtome, which should be kept well oiled during use. Slides are carefully fitted at the factory for the use of this type of oil; lubricating with oil of a different body may change the adjustment and reduce the precision of the instrument. Ordinary sewing machine and household oils are not satisfactory substitutes and are sometimes acid and corrosive. The inclined plane on the Spencer paraffin microtome No. 820 should be greased occasionally with a light neutral grease (Mobilgrease No. 1). After use all parts of the microtome should be cleaned, dried, and oiled, and the microtome protected by some type of cover. If at all possible technologists should have and be responsible for their own microtomes.

REF. Richards, O.W., "The Effective Use and Proper Care of the Microtome," American Optical Col,, 1959.

MICROSLIDES AND COVER GLASSES

Valuable technical time can be saved by purchasing precleaned, noncorrosive microslides. These are supplied in the standard 3 x 1 in. size for general use; 3 x 1 1/2 and 3 x 2 in. sizes are available for larger sections. For identification purposes, slides with a frosted marking area on one end are convenient; the plain variety can be etched with a diamond pencil. Some breakage may occur during staining. Glass marking inks are also recommended. Slides should be handled by their edges,

*Bear Oil, formerly called Pike Oil, Behr-Manning Co., Troy, N. Y.

since fingerprints leave greasy films, resulting in the
loss of sections during staining. Dirty slides must be
washed with a good detergent, rinsed well in running
tap water, passed through acid alcohol or 1% aqueous
acetic acid, and finally polished with a lint-free cloth.
They can then be stored in clean slide boxes until ready
for use.

Cover glasses come in the form of squares, rectangles,
and circles, and there is a variety of larger sizes for
special application. **Thickness of the squares varies**
from 12 to 25 mm, rectangles are 22 to 24 mm in width
and 30, 40, 50, 60 mm in length. For routine work we use
thickness No. 1 - 24 x 40 and 24 x 50 mm. Cover glasses
are sold by the ounce, and no saving is gained by purchasing thicker glasses unless they are needed for a
specific purpose. They fracture very easily and should
be handled carefully by the edges. Good-quality cover
glasses are fairly clean, but attract lint; water will
form droplets on dirty glass instead of spreading evenly.

HYDRATION OF PARAFFIN SECTIONS

Before processing sections through the various coloring
agents, residual paraffin must be removed; the customary
solvent is xylene. Sections are then hydrated by passage
through a series of alcohols of decreasing strength. If
the staining solution is alcoholic it is necessary to
hydrate only to the strength of the solution, unless
mercury crystals or other pigments must be removed.

Because the majority of tissue sections are first
stained by a general survey method such as hematoxylin
and eosin, it is convenient to have a permanent setup of
staining dishes with removal glass or metal racks. When
processing multiple sections, the slides should be stacked in the racks in such a manner that the tissue faces in
the same direction; in this way when slides are removed
to check staining or when mounting cover glasses, the
tissue side of the slide will face the technician.
This reduces the possibility of wiping the **tissue off the**
slide. Coplin jars, which holds five slides, are convenient to process special stains that require individual
differentiation.

METHOD

1. Xylene, three changes, 3 to 5 minutes.
2. Absolute alcohol, three changes 3 to 5 minutes.

3.   95% alcohol, two changes, 3 to 5 minutes.
4.   80% alcohol, one change, 3 to 5 minutes.
5.   Water.

The solutions should be replaced as necessary. Do not
allow slides to dry at any time during hydration.

   The slide washing system consists of an 18 x 12 in.
stainless steel pan, 2 1/2 in. deep, which is placed on
a Woll* drain dissecting tray near a cold water outlet
and drains into the sink. To eliminate foreign matter
the wash water is passed through a filter unit with re-
placeable cartridge and connected to the pan with rubber
tubing. The cartridge is replaced as necessary.

*Woll dissecting tray, Lipshaw Manufacturing Co., Detroit,
 Mich.

Chapter 7

NITROCELLULOSE METHOD

Since the introduction of paraffin by Klebs in 1869 as a
rapid medium for embedding, celloidin has fallen somewhat
into disuse for routine sections. It is still preferred
for the processing of eyes and for many of the procedures
used to demonstrate certain elements of the central nervous system.

The advantages of the celloidin method are that (1)
large sections can be cut, (2) it gives good support to
brittle tissue such as bone, and (3) shrinkage due to heat
is avoided. The disadvantages are that (1) sections
smaller than 15 microns are not practical, (2) the method
is time consuming, and (3) the procedure is expensive.

Celloidin is supplied in strips under the trade name
of Parlodion* (pyroxylin purified). For routine purposes
the strips are dissolved in equal parts of ether and absolute alcohol, 4% for infiltration and 8 to 12% for embedding. Large wide-mouth glass jars with screw caps
make inexpensive containers in which to dissolve celloidin. Because the solutions are viscous, jars should be in-
verted occasionally or placed on a mechanical agitator.
A magnetic stirrer (without heat) and a 500 to 1000 ml
screw-cap Erlenmeyer flask can also be used for this purpose. Stock solutions should be prepared in advance and
stored in well-stoppered wide-mouth jars, to prevent evaporation, and in the dark, since celloidin deteriorates
on exposure to light. A superior embedding material which
permits rapid infiltration and thinner sections to be cut
is called low-viscosity nitrocellulose†, tissue-embedding
solution No. 4700.

Note. The room in which celloidin work is carried out
should be free from open flame at all times.

*Parlodion (pyroxylin purified), Mallinckrodt Chemical
 Works, St. Louis, Mo.
†Randolph Products Co., Carlstadt, N. J.

DEHYDRATION AND INFILTRATION

The time required to complete dehydration varies with the
thickness of tissue blocks. The times given below are
for blocks about 4 mm thick. Infiltration time must be
increased if the tissue has been mordanted.

1. Any fixative may be used.
2. Wash tissue overnight unless otherwise indicated.
3. 70% alcohol, two changes, 24 hours.
4. 80% alcohol, two changes, 24 hours.
5. 95% alcohol, two changes, 24 hours.
6. Absolute alcohol, two changes, 24 hours.
7. Absolute alcohol and ether, equal parts, two changes,
   24 hours.
8. Infiltrate tissue in thin celloidin in a well-covered
   dish for 1 week.
9. Transfer tissue to embedding dish in 8% to 12%
   celloidin.

EMBEDDING

Square staining dishes without grooves, or Stender dishes
with ground glass covers, are suitable containers. Dishes
with concave or convex bottoms should not be used. The
pressure of evaporated celloidin will cause the section
to bow and take on the shape of the dish. This represents
the cutting surface and many sections will be lost in
trimming. The volume of celloidin should be sufficient
to allow evaporation without exposing the upper surface
of the tissue block. As evaporation progresses, celloidin
will cling to the sides of the dish and become concave in
the center.
     Place the tissue in the embedding dish with the sur-
face to be sectioned facedown, taking care not to introduce air bubbles into the celloidin. Keep the dish covered for 1 to 2 days to permit any air that may have been
trapped to escape and raise the cover for a few hours
each day to evaporate the ether alcohol.
     An alternate method is to place the dish under a bell
jar or in a desiccator and after 1 to 2 days to allow the
solution to thicken by raising the bell jar or sliding
the lid to one side of the desiccator for a short period
each day; do not leave the embedding jars uncovered overnight. If the cover is left off for too long a period,
a hard skin will form on the top of the celloidin, pre-
venting evaporation, while the fluid below remains soft.
If this happens, pour a little ether alcohol solution into

the dish and replace the cover; the skin will dissolve.
Evaporation should proceed so that the consistency of the
whole block will be uniform.

We have used vacuum to reduce the time necessary for
infiltration and to remove trapped air, by placing the
specimen in thin celloidin in a tall glass jar in the
vacuum oven without heat at about 10 to 15 mm of Hg.
Thin celloidin is added as necessary; at night the jar is
removed from the vacuum and covered. Small specimens may
be infiltrated in 2 to 3 days by this method.

After the celloidin has solidified to the consistency
of soft rubber and can just be indented with a fingernail,
run a sharp blade around the inside of the embedding dish
to free the celloidin from the sides.

This will allow ether alcohol to evaporate further
and will prevent the celloidin from sinking in the middle.
The hardening procedure may be accelerated by placing a
small amount of chloroform in an open dish under the bell
jar or in the desiccator.

When the celloidin has the same consistency throughout, remove it carefully from the dish and place the block
overnight in 70% alcohol; the block will harden in a few
hours if a little chloroform is added to the alcohol. No
attempt should be made to remove the celloidin mass from
the dish until it is firm enough; otherwise the tissue
will remain attached to the bottom of the dish.

When the celloidin has a firm consistency throughout,
trim off the excess with a sharp knife, making all sides
parallel and leaving a small margin of celloidin around
the specimen; the mounting surface should be absolutely
flat.

MOUNTING

Grooved Phenolic Resin blocks, slightly larger than the
base of the celloidin block, make suitable holders. Wood-
en blocks are not recommended, because the resins in the
wood discolor alcohols and tissue during storage. To attach the celloidin block to the fiber block, allow the
celloidin block to remain exposed to the air for 15 to 20
minutes to evaporate the surface alcohol. Using two Petri
dishes, one containing ether alcohol and the other 8 to
12% celloidin, dip the mounting surface of the celloidin
block for a minute or so into the ether alcohol, then both
blocks into the thick celloidin, and gently press the two
blocks together, with the celloidin block uppermost.
While holding the blocks firmly in place with the thumb
and index fingers, spread excess celloidin with a spatula
so that it adheres to the sides of the celloidin block;

the whole mass should be free of air bubbles and opaque
areas between the mounting surfaces.
     Expose the block to the air for 5 to 10 minutes, then
place in 70% alcohol overnight. If time is short, place
the block in chloroform vapors in a bell jar to set the
celloidin; it is then ready for sectioning. Blocks and
cut sections may be stored indefinitely in 70% alcohol.
To discard used liquid celloidin, pour the solution into
a dish pan of cold water, remove when solid, and then discard in a container.

SECTION CUTTING

A variety of foreign and domestic microtomes are available to section celloidin-embedded material. Large immersion floor models are used to section whole organs;
smaller types, either base sledge or sliding, are used
for tissue sections. On the larger microtome, the knife
is stationary, while the tissue block moves; on the small
er model, the action is reversed. Some are adaptable
for larger frozen or paraffin sections that cannot be
accommodated on rotary-type microtomes. Because celloidin offers more resistance to sectioning than paraffin,
in our experience a microtome that permits the knife to
be clamped at both ends is preferable.
     Knives used for celloidin work may be wedge shaped or
planoconcave. We prefer the former. The latter type of
knife should be inserted into the knife holder with its
plane side toward the block. Celloidin knives require a
sharp edge free from serrations; any irregularities on
the knife edge will show up on the section. The knife is
set in the holder as obliquely as possible so that most
of the cutting edge will be used when sectioning. The
tilt of the knife will depend on the hardness of the material being sectioned. Normally the tilt will be greater than that used for cutting paraffin sections; if not,
incomplete sections will result.
     The block and knife edge should be kept moist with
70% alcohol, either with a drip apparatus or absorbent
cotton. The block is trimmed until a full section is obtained. All adjustments to the knife and microtome should
be complete at this point. The tissue block and knife
should be kept dust-free, since particles on the surface
of the block or knife edge will spoil the section.
     Sections are usually cut at 15 to 20 microns. Tissue
cut to less than a 15-micron thickness has a tendency to
curl; uncurl the section by stroking it up the knife with
a camel's hair brush before proceeding to cut a full section. When sectioning, do not pause when the knife is in

contact with the tissue, since this will cause a ridge to form.

Sections may be transferred to 70% alcohol with fine forceps or flattened out on the knife with a camel's hair brush moistened with 70% alcohol. Then with a piece of cigarette or onion-skin paper moistened with 70% alcohol placed on the section, it can be lifted from the knife and put in alcohol; the paper should be slightly larger than the celloidin block.

Celloidin is a nonribboning material; when cutting serial sections, the papers are numbered and placed in order between sections. Serial sections should be cut as rapidly as possible without too much time lapse between cuts; otherwise evaporation may cause shrinkage of the celloidin, resulting in lost or uneven sections.

STAINING

Most routine staining methods are applicable to celloidin sections. To obtain a delicate stain on thick sections, the staining solution should be diluted with distilled water and, because the dye has to penetrate the celloidin film, the staining time prolonged. Unmounted sections are usually carried through the various reagents and mounted on microslides without removing the celloidin; in the final preparation the celloidin should be colorless.

Petri or Pyrex baking dishes can be used for staining, depending on the size of the sections, which can be carried through the solutions with a glass "hockey stick" or a section lifter.

Sections can be mounted before staining by the following method. Transfer sections from 70 to 95% alcohol, mount on microslide and blot with a fine filter paper, dip in 0.5% celloidin for a few seconds, drain and wipe the back of the slide, place in chloroform to harden the celloidin film, rinse in 95% alcohol, and then place in 70% alcohol until ready to stain.

DEHYDRATION AND CLEARING

Absolute alcohol should not be used to dehydrate sections; the celloidin will soften or dissolve completely, as well as wrinkle, and the section will not flatten out in the clearing fluid. When mounted on slides, wrinkles tend to fold and trap air bubbles, which cannot be removed; for this reason essential oils such as bergamot, thyme oil, cedarwood, and terpineol which clear from 95% alcohol must be used. Because of its adverse action on many of the coal tar dyes, clearing solutions containing phenol (carbolic acid) should be avoided. Certain methods such as Weigert-Pal or Marchi are not affected by phenol.

When mounting, celloidin is retained; the mounting media should be more viscous than usual. Cover glasses of No. 2 thickness are recommended for large sections and should be slightly smaller than the slide. After the section is mounted and the slide carefully wiped free of mounting media, it is placed on a flat surface, a clean lead weight is placed on the cover glass, and the slide is allowed to dry overnight at room temperature; a final cleaning is given the following day.

Baker recommends the following sequence to dehydrate and clear celloidin sections.

1. Place sections in 90% alcohol.
2. Absolute alcohol and chloroform, equal parts, 1 to 2 minutes.
3. Absolute alcohol, chloroform, and xylene, equal parts, 1 to 2 minutes.
4. Xylene, two changes until cleared.

OTHER METHODS OF DEHYDRATION AND CLEARING

A. 1. 70% alcohol
    2. Aniline oil.
    3. Xylene, three changes or until oil is removed.
    4. Mount.

B. 1. 95% alcohol.
    2. Weigert's carbol-xylene.

        Carbolic acid   1 part
        Xylene   3 parts

    3. Xylene, two changes.
    4. Mount.

C. 1. 95% alcohol.
    2. Terpineol until section sinks.
    3. Xylene, two changes.
    4. Mount.

RAPID CELLOIDIN EMBEDDING METHOD FOR THIN SECTIONS ONLY

Fixation. 10% formalin or Carnoy's fluid.

1. Wash formalin-fixed tissue in tap water; Carnoy's fixed material is processed without washing.

2.	95% alcohol, 1 hour.	8 a.m.
3.	95% alcohol, 1 hour.	9 a.m.
4.	95% alcohol, 1 hour.	10 a.m.
5.	Absolute alcohol, 1 hour.	11 a.m.
6.	Absolute alcohol, 1 hour.	12 p.m.
7.	Absolute alcohol and ether, equal parts, 1 hour.	1 p.m.
8.	Absolute alcohol and ether, equal parts, 1 hour.	2 p.m.
9.	Thin celloidin, 2 hours.	3 p.m.
10.	Thick celloidin, 15 hours.	5 p.m.

At 8 a.m., the following morning, mount on fiber block (tissue is not embedded in a solid block of celloidin), cover the mass with thick celloidin, allow to dry for a few minutes in the air, then harden in chloroform if needed immediately. Sections may be cut off after 2 to 3 hours, or stored in 70% alcohol and cut the following day.

ACETONE CELLOIDIN (Rapid method for small specimens only)

Fixation. Carnoy's fluid.

1. Rinse in two to three changes of absolute alcohol to remove chloroform.
2. Acetone, 2 hours.
3. Acetone, 2 hours.
4. Thin celloidin, 2 hours.
5. Thick celloidin, 2 hours.

Place the tissue on a fiber block carrying over excess celloidin, allow to air-dry until a film has formed, then complete hardening in chloroform or 70% alcohol.

BARRON'S AMYL ACETATE METHOD

The following procedure was used to process a formalin fixed puppy brain in toto.

1. Acetone, 48 hours.
2. Acetone and amyl acetate, half and half, 48 hours.
3. Amyl acetate, 24 hours.
4. 2% celloidin in amyl acetate, 24 hours.
5. 6% celloidin in amyl acetate, 24 hours.
6. 12% celloidin in amyl acetate, 24 hours.
7. Embed in thick celloidin, 24 hours.

Ref.   Barron, D. H., Anat. Record, 59, 1 (1934).

Chapter 8

ACCESSORY PROCEDURES TO STAINING

REMOVAL OF MERCURY CRYSTALS

If sections are Zenker or Helly (Zenker-formal) fixed or if the fixative contains mercuric chloride, remove the crystals as follows:

LUGOL'S IODINE (LANGERON)

Iodine crystals	1 gm
Potassium iodide	2 gm
Distilled water	200 ml

Dissolve the potassium iodide in a small amount of water, add the iodine and shake to dissolve, and then add the balance of the water.

1. Lugol's iodine, 3 to 5 minutes.
2. Wash in running water, 3 to 5 minutes.
3. 5% aqueous sodium thiosulfate, 3 to 5 minutes.
4. Wash in running water, 5 minutes.

R. Gonzales [Stain Tech., **34**, 2, (1959)] recommends the following procedure to simultaneously dehydrate and remove mercury crystals.

1. Fix the tissue for the required time.
2. Wash in water or immerse directly in cellosolve (ethylene glycol monoethyl ether). Leave for 24 to 48 hours in three changes.
3. Clear in benzene or xylene for 1 to 2 hours.
4. Infiltrate and embed in paraffin.

REMOVAL OF PICRIC ACID STAINS

The yellow stain from picric acid in Bouin's or other fixatives containing it can be removed by inserting a bath of saturated lithium carbonate (3 gm) in 70% alcohol in the hydration series after the last alcohol; the sections are left for 2 minutes and then washed in water.

Gray recommends Lenoir's fluid.

LENOIR'S FLUID

Distilled water	70 ml
95% alcohol	30 ml
Ammonium acetate	10 gm

Ref.   Gary, P., Handbook of Basic Microtechnique, 3rd ed. Used with permission of McGraw-Hill Book Co., N. Y.

REMOVAL OF PIGMENTS

Formalin Pigment

Saturate solution of picric acid (9 gm) in absolute alcohol for 1 to 2 hours, wash well in tap water. This does not remove melanin pigments.

Melanin

1.   0.25% aqueous potassium permanganate for 12 to 24 hours. Wash in water for 5 minutes. 1% aqueous oxalic acid for 1 minute. Wash in water for 5 to 10 minutes.
2.   10% aqueous hydrogen peroxide for 24 to 48 hours. Wash well in water.
3.   1% aqueous chromic acid and 5% calcium chloride, in equal parts, for 8 to 12 hours. Wash well in water.

Malaria

1.   3% aqueous hydrogen peroxide for 2 to 3 hours. Wash well in water.
2.   Acetone   50 ml
       Hydrogen peroxide, 3%   50 ml
       Ammonium hydroxide, 28%   1 ml
       Place deparaffinized sections in solution for 1 hour or more, then wash well in water.
3.   Saturated solution of picric acid in absolute alcohol (9 gm) for 1 to 24 hours. Wash well in water.

LENDRUM'S TAMP METHOD FOR IMPROVING STAINING
OF INADEQUATELY FIXED TISSUE

1.   Deparaffinize sections.
2.   Rinse well in absolute alcohol.
3.   Transfer directly to the following solution for 24 to
      48 hours in a closed container.
      Trichloroethylene   250 ml
      Saturated picric acid in absolute
      alcohol (about 9%)   250 ml
      Mercuric chloride   5 gm
4.   Rinse in absolute alcohol.
5.   Rinse in 80% alcohol.
6.   Place in 0.5% iodine in 70% alcohol for 5 minutes.
7.   Wash in water.
8.   Place in 2% sodium thiosulfate for 5 minutes.
9.   Wash in tap water long enough to remove the picric
      acid. The section is now ready for staining. Most,
      but not all, staining gives improved results after
      this pretreatment.

Note. This procedure improves the staining of sections
      from tissue that have been inadequately fixed, and
      to remove the formalin deposit that occurs in rela-
      tion to erythrocytes, which may be present in amounts
      sufficient to upset silver methods for reticulin or
      to render staining of erythrocytes rather dull.

Ref. Personal communication.

POSTMORDANTING

At times it is necessary to pretreat tissue received in
other fixatives in order to obtain the desired staining
results. The usual procedure is to place deparaffinized
sections in the fixative called for. In the case of
Helly's or Zenker's fluids, a saturated aqueous solution
of mercuric chloride for 5 to 10 minutes will provide the
necessary mordanting; as usual, the mercury crystals will
have to be removed before staining. Bouin's fixative may
be replaced by a saturated solution of picric acid in
absolute alcohol for 5 to 10 minutes; wash sections well
in water before staining. Remove yellow stain of picric
acid by immersing sections in a saturated solution of
lithium carbonate (3 gm) in 70% alcohol for 2 to 3 minutes. Wash in water.

DESTAINING AND RESTAINING

Faded slides may be restained by the same or by a different method by soaking off the cover glass in xylene at room temperature or in a 60°C oven in a covered dish. The time varies depending on the age of the slide; do not try to force the cover glass off, since this may damage the section. Another method, which requires some skill, is to gently heat the bottom of the slide over a Bunsen burner (the slide should not become uncomfortable to the touch); when bubbles appear in the mounting media, place the slide in xylene and the cover glass will float off. Place the slide in fresh xylene to remove all old mounting medium, then in absolute alcohol, 95% alcohol, and water. Remove the old stain in acid alcohol, rinse well in water, and restain. Slides may also be decolorized in 0.5% aqueous potassium permanganate for 5 minutes, rinsed in water for 5 minutes, bleached in 0.5% aqueous oxalic acid for 5 minutes, then washed in water and restained. Caution should be exercised in the interpretation of iron stains on sections previously stained in iron hematoxylin solutions.

   If more than one section is mounted on a slide, and the original stain must be preserved, gently score the cover glass with a diamond pencil, using another slide as a guide. Place the slide in a Coplin jar in xylene just sufficient to cover the score, without disturbing the remaining cover glass. When the section is exposed, rinse away excess mounting media with fresh xylene. Place the slide in a small volume of absolute alcohol, rinse in water, and destain and restain as desired. Dehydrate; the remaining cover glass can be removed in xylene and the slide remounted.

CELLOIDIN COATING OF LOOSE SECTIONS

If it is suspected that sections may loosen or float off slides during staining because of one of the following conditions--inadequate fixation, alkaline or acid staining solutions, excess soaking before sectioning, prestained tissue to be restained and brittle tissue--the sections can be coated with a thin film of celloidin before staining as follows. Remove paraffin with xylene and place in absolute alcohol. Place sections in a 0.05% solution of celloidin dissolved in equal parts of ether and absolute alcohol. Drain excess celloidin and air-dry briefly, and then place in 70% alcohol to harden celloidin. Wash in water and stain as desired. The celloidin film will be removed during dehydration in absolute alcohol.

A METHOD FOR SALVAGING HISTOLOGICAL SECTIONS FROM BROKEN MICROSLIDES

Glass Jig

A 3 1/2 x 4 in. lantern slide is used as a base. Two 1 x 3 in. microslides, shimmed by one or more 22 x 40 mm cover glasses, are cemented (with household cement) along the shorter edge of the base. These serve as guides to a 5-in. length of 12-mm (outside diameter) glass tubing, which is used to smooth the coating material. The thickness of the film produced is determined by the number of cover glasses used as shims. The thickness of the cemented microslide-cover glass guide should exceed that of the slide to be repaired by at least one No. 1 cover glass.

Coating Material

Cyclon-Lack farbols No. 10830, lufttocknend[*]. We have used Diatex[†] with good results.

PROCEDURE

1. Remove broken cover glass by soaking in xylene. Remove label.
2. While it is still wet with xylene, place the slide in the jig section side up.
3. Place a large drop of coating material next to the section and spread it with the glass tubing.
4. Dry the coated slide in a 57°C oven for 1 hour.
5. Place slide in cool water for 2 to 3 hours to loosen film.
6. Carefully strip film containing section from slide.
7. Dry film carefully between filter paper.
8. Trim away excess film, place on fresh slide, and cover glass in Permount.

Ref. Geil, R. G., Tech. Bull. Reg. Med. Tech., __31__, 195-196 (1961).
Weibel used the same plastic in his film-stripping technique.

[*]Cyclon-Lack farbols No. 10830, lufttrocknend.
 Thinner: Cyclon-Lack Verduennung L+.
[†]Diate Mounting Media, Scientific Products

Chapter 9

DYES AND STAINING

The art of dyeing fabrics dates back to 3000 B.C. The
Greeks and Romans were highly skilled in the use of natural dyes obtained from animal or vegetable sources. Dio-
scorides, the Greek physician, described many dye plants,
and the Roman naturalist, Pliny the Elder, outlined the
preparation of dyes from certain shellfish, which was the
source of the famous Tyrian purple.

Cochineal was introduced into Europe by the Spanish
who brought it from New Spain, now Mexico; it is obtained
from the dried bodies of the female insect "Dactylopius
Cacti." Carminic acid is obtained from cochineal and was
an important dye to the early histologist; it is still
used to demonstrate glycogen. Maddar, a vegetable dye obtained from the roots of the Maddar plant, yields various
shades of red. This dye has been used to demonstrate the
development of growing bone in young animals; alizarin,
one of the products of Maddar, is now produced synthet-
ically.

One of the most important natural dyes for use in
histology is hematoxylin, which comes from a leguminous
tree that grows wild along the coast of Mexico and South
America. The heartwood or logwood is red-tinted orange
and black; the coloring substance prepared from logwood
is haematein. Hematoxylin was first introduced into Europe in the sixteenth century by Francisco Hernandez,
court physician to Philip II of Spain, who was the first
person to describe its staining properties.

Except for natural or artificial pigments, unstained
tissue elements do not present enough contrast to be
examined under the bright-field microscope; staining ren-
ders the tissue components more visible, usually in contrasting colors. Leeuwenhoek, in 1714, was the first to
use natural dyes in studying muscle.

Chemical or artificial dyestuffs assumed great importance with the discovery of the aniline color mauve by
William Perkins in 1856. The discovery of various other
dyes followed rapidly, and at present there are several
thousand organic dyes available. Their use in histology

71

was first described by Bencke in 1862. Dr. Joseph Wood-
ward (1833-1884), a member of the original staff of the
Army Medical Museum, was the first in the United States
to stain histological sections with aniline dyes.

The first artificial dyes were produced from aniline,
and were called "aniline dyes." Today most dyes are manu-
factured from coal tar and may be considered as deriva-
tives of the hydrocarbon benzene.

The first artificial dyes used by microscopists were
crude textile dyes, and results were not always reproducible. The Dr. G. Grubler Co. was formed in Germany not
to manufacture dyes, but to test dyes suitable for biological purposes; the methods of standardization were empirical, and dyes varied in composition from batch to
batch. Nevertheless, Grubler dyes were the best available and were used throughout the world before World War I.

During the war the German dye supply was cut off;
available dyes were contaminated and became unsuitable for
biological purposes. This situation led to the organization in the United States of the Commission on Standardization of Biological Stains under the direction of H. J.
Conn. The organization is now known as The Biological
Stain Commission. Its function is to test dyes submitted
by manufacturers to be sold as biological stains.

A special label is furnished to a submitting company
by the commission for each batch of dye tested; at a
slight additional cost dyes so tested can be obtained with
the commission's certification number on the label. In-
formation about these dyes is available in the quarterly
lists published in the Stain Commission journal "Stain
Technology."

Because of the great number of synonyms attached to
dyes by various manufacturers, it is advisable when purchasing dyes to give the Color Index Number (C. I. No.) of
the desired dye. The total dye content varies from batch
to batch, as indicated on the label; this should be taken
into consideration when staining, increasing or decreasing the time as necessary.

Dyes are expensive and should be stored carefully to
avoid deterioration. Warm or damp places should be avoided; the storage cupboard should be away from direct sunlight. Dry stains will keep indefinitely if the bottles
are well stoppered, acids and ammonium hydroxide should
not be stored near them. Stains in solution should be
treated in a like manner and are best kept in glass-stop-
pered brown bottles. Some aqueous dye solutions support
the growth of molds; this can be prevented by the addition
of a few drops of chloroform or a crystal of thymol.

Distilled water used to make up dye solutions should
be fresh, since stale distilled water absorbs carbon di-

oxide, which produces an acid reaction that may interfere with certain staining procedures such as Giemsa or methyl green-pyronin. This condition can sometimes be corrected by boiling the water before use. Acids and ammonium hydroxide should not be stored near the distilled water supply.

Some staining solutions deteriorate spontaneously, so that the date on which the solution is prepared should be noted on the label. It is good practice to filter stain solutions before use to check if precipitates are forming. Staining solutions used to demonstrate bacteria should always be filtered.

THEORY OF STAINING

The staining of tissue elements and pathological products in different colors depends on a variety of conditions, which are not fully understood. In the past the chemical and physical theories held sway, but, as Conn points out, "Most of this controversy is now distinctly out of date, as it has become evident that physiochemical phenomena are involved which operate in the borderland between more obvious physical and chemical reactions."

The physical theory held that the dye penetrated the tissue by osmosis or capillary force, by adsorption or absorption and diffusion, or by precipitation by acids and bases. The chemical theory held that the dye had certain affinities for some portion of the protoplasm. It was assumed that certain parts of the cell such as the nuclei were acid and had an affinity for basic dyes and that the cytoplasm was basic in character and therefore had an affinity for acid dyes. Most staining procedures are complex and are not as easily explained as the iron reaction in which ferric iron combines with potassium ferrocyanide to form ferric ferrocyanide, producing a blue color called "Prussian blue." Lipid stains are considered physical in reaction in which oil-soluble dyes have a greater affinity for lipids in tissue than the solvent in which they are dissolved.

No one dye or staining procedure will demonstrate all tissue elements. Most procedures combine two or more dyes mixed together or in such a sequence that the various tissue elements are outlined in contrasting colors--this is known as differential staining. The term metachromophil is applied to a substance not reacting normally to staining.

In general, dyes stain orthochromatically, that is, a blue dye will stain blue and a red dye red. Certain basic triarylmethane dyes such as methyl violet or crystal

violet, and especially dyes of the thiazine group such as
methylene blue or thionin, stain metachromatically when
applied from an aqueous solution. In reality the dye
exists in two distinct forms,--the normal color blue and
the metachromatic color red. Because of this character-
istic, certain tissue elements will stain blue and others
in shades from red to purple. The metachromatic reaction
is not a result of impurities in the dye but is due to
various sulfuric esters present in mucin, mast cell granules, or the ground substance of cartilage, which are
capable of altering the color of a metachromatic dye,
thereby taking up the red component of the dye. These
substances are termed chromotrophic. This specified reaction proves useful to demonstrate these substances his-
tochemically.
     Unfortunately, metachromasia is almost or completely
lost in the process of dehydration in absolute alcohol or
other reagents used for this purpose. It can be preserved
fairly well in some types of aqueous mounting media as potassium acetate, or the commercial product Valnor, less
so in glycerin jelly, which is slightly acidic
     In our experience, unfixed cryostat sectioning is the
method of choice to demonstrate metachromasia, notably in
amyloid. Staining of identical, formalin-fixed, paraffin-
embedded material appears rather dull in comparison. When
observing metachromatic substances microscopically, the
blue glass filter should be removed.

METHODS OF STAINING

Progressive Staining

The tissue elements are stained up to a point; staining
is stopped when the desired intensity has been reached.
The degree of staining is controlled with the microscope.
This type of staining requires no differentiation.

Regressive Staining

The tissue is deliberately overstained, and the excess dye
is washed out in a suitable solution until the correct degree of color intensity is attained. Alcohol, acid alcohol, another dye, or in some cases the mordant are used
as differentiating fluids. At times differentiation with
alcohols is combined with the dehydration sequence.

Direct or Substantive Staining

The dye attaches itself directly to some tissue component;
no mordant is required. The dye is withdrawn from the

solution by the tissue and confers upon the latter a
depth of color depending on the strength of the solution
and the affinity of the tissue for the dye.

Indirect or Adjective Staining

Many dyes do not have direct affinity for tissue elements;
mordants (L. mordere--to bite) act as binders between dye
and tissue elements, operating on the principle that the
tissue is first impregnated with a chemical capable of
attaching itself to the tissue and subsequently to the
dye. The resulting compound is called a lake, which is
usually insoluble in neutral solutions used in microtechnique allowing many complex staining procedures to be
carried out. Mordants were known and used around 2000 B.C.
to dye textiles and to stabilize colors of natural dyes.
Progressive, regressive, and mordant are terms acquired
from the dyeing industry.
    Mordants are salts of metals such as aluminum and
ammonium sulfate, aluminum and potassium sulfate, and
ferric and ammonium sulfate, to name a few that are commonly used with hematoxylin, producing colors from blue
to black. Certain staining procedures require a particular fixative containing the necessary mordant to bring
about a specific reaction between dye and tissue, such as
Zenker or Helly's fluids for Mallory's phosphotungstic
acid hematoxylin stain.
    Mordants may be used prior to staining or be included
in the dye solution. Usually regressive staining relies
on the use of mordants; acid alcohol, or the mordant itself is generally used to differentiate the excess dye
from unwanted areas in the tissue.
    Accentuators should not be confused with mordants;
these substances, which enhance the action of dyes on
tissue, do not become part of the lake. They increase
the staining power or selectivity of the dye without chemical combination. (Example: phenol in carbol thionin or
carbol fuchsin, or borax in methylene blue.) Ramon Cajal
termed certain hypnotics (chloral hydrate or nicotene)
accelerators; these substances are used in the metallic
methods to demonstrate elements of the central nervous
system.
    It should be noted that the times given in staining
procedures usually are approximate and must be varied to
meet requirements of a particular fixative or tissue.
There is no exact method for predetermining the time required to stain a particular tissue component; practical
experience with various staining procedures is the best
guide.
    When staining in bulk, such as hematoxylin and eosin,

representative sections should be checked under the
microscope to control differentiation. The same applies
to counterstaining with eosin.
     Before starting a procedure read it through, check
the time required to complete the method, and see that
all the necessary solutions are on hand.

HEMATOXYLIN SOLUTIONS

When pure, hematoxylin forms nearly colorless crystals
which are not a dye, but an oxidation commonly referred
to as ripening. Hematoxylin is converted into the color
substance haematein which forms colored lakes with various mordants. This process of oxidation may be carried
out in solution and speeded up by the addition of different oxidizing agents, such as potassium permanganate or
sodium iodate.
     Mallory lists various metals that, when combined with
hematoxylin or applied as mordants, will demonstrate various tissue components.

Aluminum, iron, tungsten	Nuclei
Chromium, copper, iron	Myelin sheaths
Iron (also iodine)	Elastic fibers
Molybdenum	Collagen
Tungsten	Fibroglia, myoglia, neu-roglia, epithelial fibers, and fibrin
Lead	Axis cylinders
Iron	Mucin

AQUEOUS ALUM HEMATOXYLIN

Hematoxylin crystals	1 gm
Aluminum and ammonium sulfate (ammonia alum)	20 gm
Distilled water	400 ml
Thymol	1 gm

Dissolve the hematoxylin in 100 ml of distilled water with
the aid of heat and add the alum dissolved in the balance
of the distilled water. Add the thymol to prevent the
growth of mold. Expose the solution to light and air in
a lightly stoppered flask (cotton plug). The solution
will ripen in about 10 days, after which it should be kept
in a tightly stoppered bottle; the solution lasts for 2
to 3 months.

BENNETT'S HEMATOXYLIN

Distilled water (hot)	1000 ml
Hematoxylin crystals	1 gm
Sodium iodate	0.2 gm
Aluminum and potassium sulfate (potassium alum)	90 gm
Chloral hydrate	50 gm
Citric acid	1 gm

Add the ingredients successively, dissolving each in turn. Can be used immediately; lasts for months.

BULLARD'S HEMATOXYLIN

Ethyl alcohol, 50%	144 ml
Glacial acetic acid	16 ml
Hematoxylin crystals	8 gm
Heat and add:	
Distilled water	250 ml
Aluminum and ammonium sulfate (ammonia alum)	20 gm
Heat to boiling, slowly and carefully add:	
Mercuric oxide red	8 gm
Cool quickly, filter, and add:	
Ethyl alcohol, 95%	275 ml
Glycerin	330 ml
Glacial acetic acid	18 ml
Aluminum and ammonium sulfate (ammonia alum)	40 gm

Solution lasts for a year or more; may be used immediately.

DELAFIELD'S HEMATOXYLIN

Hematoxylin crystals	4 gm
Ethyl alcohol, 95%	24 ml
Saturated aqueous solution of aluminum and ammonium sulfate Approximately 45 gm (ammonia alum)	400 ml

Add the hematoxylin dissolved in the alcohol to the alum solution and expose the mixture in an unstoppered bottle to light and air for 2 to 4 days.

EHRLICH'S ACID HEMATOXYLIN

Hematoxylin crystals   6 gm
Absolute ethyl alcohol   300 ml
Dissolve in water bath and filter:
Glycerin   300 ml
Distilled water   300 ml
Glacial acetic acid   30 ml
Aluminum and potassium sulfate
(potassium alum) to excess   About 40 gm

Add the ingredients in the order given, mix thoroughly,
and expose to light for 6 weeks to ripen. Solution lasts
for years.

Baker and Jordan's method of oxidizing: Add 0.3 gm of
sodium iodate to solution without acetic acid. Bring to
a boil, cool, add acetic acid, and filter. The solution
is ready for use.

HARRIS' HEMATOXYLIN

Hematoxylin crystals   5 gm
Absolute ethyl alcohol   50 ml
Aluminum and potassium sulfate
(potassium alum)   100 gm
Mercuric oxide (red)   2.5 gm
Distilled water   1000 ml

Dissolve the hematoxylin in the alcohol and the alum in
the water with the aid of heat. Mix the two solutions
together and bring to a boil. Withdraw the flame, slowly
and carefully add the mercuric oxide, heat gently, and
allow to continue to boil for 5 minutes. Place the flask
in cold water and cool quickly. Filter and add 40 ml of
glacial acetic acid to improve nuclear staining. Filter
solution each time before use; solution is effective for
1 to 2 months.

HEIDENHAIN'S IRON HEMATOXYLIN

Hematoxylin crystals   0.5 gm
Absolute ethyl alcohol   10 ml
Distilled water   90 ml

Dissolve the hematoxylin in the alcohol and add the distilled water. Place in a cotton-plugged flask and allow
to ripen for 4 to 5 weeks. For use dilute with equal
parts of distilled water; the solution may be used repeatedly.

Or: 5% alcoholic solution of hema-
    toxylin (well ripened)   10 ml
    Distilled water   90 ml

This solution may be used immediately.

JANSSEN'S HEMATOXYLIN: GURR

Iron alum (ferric ammonium sulfate, purple crystals only), 10%·
aqueous   50 ml
10% hematoxylin in absolute alcohol 10 ml
Absolute methyl alcohol   15 ml
Glycerin   15 ml
Distilled water   20 ml

Allow solution to stand for 1 week before using.

MALLORY'S PHOSPHOTUNGSTIC ACID HEMATOXYLIN

Hematoxylin crystals   1 gm
Phosphotungstic acid   20 gm
Distilled water   1000 ml

Dissolve the hematoxylin and the phosphotungstic acid
separately in distilled water with the aid of gentle heat.
When cool, combine the solutions. To ripen immediately,
add 0.177 gm of potassium permanganate, or expose to light
for 6 to 7 weeks. Solution keeps well for months.

MAYER'S HEMALUM (Acid Alum Hematoxylin)

Hematoxylin crystals   1 gm
Sodium iodate   0.2 gm
Aluminum and ammonium sulfate
(ammonia alum)   50 gm
Chloral hydrate   50 gm
Citric acid   1 gm
Distilled water   1000 ml

Dissolve the hematoxylin in the distilled water with the
aid of gentle heat, add the sodium iodate and the ammonia
alum. When the latter is dissolved, add the citric acid
and the chloral hydrate; the solution turns a reddish
violet. The solution keeps well; when a dirty brown color
appears solution is exhausted--in approximately 2 to 3
months.

PAPAMILTIADES' HEMATOXYLIN

Hematoxylin, 1% aqueous	100 ml
Aluminum sulfate, 5% aqueous	50 ml
Zinc sulfate, 5% aqueous	25 ml
Potassium iodide, 4% aqueous	25 ml
Glacial acetic acid	8 ml
Glycerin	25 ml

Solution may be used immediately; lasts for approximately 2 months. This solution acts as a progressive stain and requires little, if any, differentiation.

Ref. Papamiltiades, M., Acta Anat., 19, 24 (1953).

REGAUD'S HEMATOXYLIN

Hematoxylin crystals	1 gm
Ethyl alcohol, 95%	10 ml
Glycerin	10 ml
Distilled water	80 ml

Allow to ripen for 3 weeks, or prepare with 10 ml of a ripened alcoholic hematoxylin solution instead of the first two solutions.

SLIDDER'S IRON HEMATOXYLIN

Hematoxylin crystals	1 gm
Ethyl alcohol, 95%	100 ml
Aluminum chloral hydrate	10 gm
Ferrous sulfate hydrate	10 gm
Distilled water	100 ml

When dissolved, combine solutions and add 2 ml of concentrated hydrochloric acid and 2 ml of 9% sodium iodate (saturate solution at 20°C). Mix and allow to stand for 48 hours; the stain is now ready for use. Keep in a 200-ml screw-cap bottle.

Ref. Slidders, W., J. Microscopy, 90:1 (1969), 61-65.

EOSIN-Y COUNTERSTAINING SOLUTIONS

ALCOHOLIC EOSIN-Y SOLUTION

Eosin-Y, 3% aqueous solution	100 ml
Absolute ethyl alcohol	125 ml
Distilled water	375 ml

AQUEOUS EOSIN-Y SOLUTION

Eosin-Y	10 gm
Distilled water	1000 ml
Glacial acetic acid	2 ml

OXALIC ACID-EOSIN-Y SOLUTION

Eosin-Y or phloxine, 1% aqueous	100 ml
Oxalic acid, 1% aqueous	5 ml

Ref. Delez, A. L. and Davis, O. S., Stain Tech., 25, 2
     (1950).

PUTT'S EOSIN-Y SOLUTION

Eosin-Y	5 gm
Potassium dichromate	2.5 gm
Saturated aqueous picric acid	
(1 to 1 1/2%)	50 ml
Absolute ethyl alcohol	50 ml
Distilled water	400 ml

Dissolve the eosin-Y in the alcohol and the potassium dichromate in distilled water, combine the two, and add the
saturated solution of picric acid. Filter.

Ref. Putt, F. A., Arch. Path., 45 (1948).

RED NUCLEAR STAINS

DARROW RED

Darrow red	50 gm
0.2M glacial acetic acid (pH 2.7)	200 ml

Heat if necessary to dissolve the dye, then filter. Lasts
about 1 month.

MAYER'S CARMALUM

Carminic acid	1 gm
Ammonium or potassium alum	10 gm
Distilled water	200 ml
Salicylic acid	0.2 gm

Dissolve with heat if necessary, cool, and add the sali-
cylic acid.

NUCLEAR FAST RED (KERNECHTROT)

Nuclear fast red (Kernechtrot)   0.1 gm
Aluminum sulfate, 5% aqueous   100 ml

Dissolve the Kernechtrot in the aluminum sulfate solution
with the aid of heat, cool and filter, then add a crystal
of thymol. Solution keeps well at room temperature and
can be reused.

SAFRANINE

Safranine   0.2 gm
Distilled water   100 ml
Glacial acetic acid   1 ml

SCARBA-RED

Melt 2 gm of phenol in a flask under hot water, add 1 gm
of neutral red, and mix thoroughly; allow the mixture to
cool and dissolve the cold sludge in 15 ml of 95% methyl
alcohol. To this add 85 ml of 2% aniline in water and 1
to 3 ml of glacial acetic acid. Mix well and filter.

Differentiator

70% ethyl alcohol   85 ml
Formalin, 40%   15 ml
Glacial acetic acid   15 drops

Ref. Slidders, W., Frazer, D. S., Smith, R. and Lendrum,
     A. C., J. Path. Bact., **75** 476-478, (1958).

BIOLOGICAL STAINS COMMONLY USED IN HISTOLOGY

A denotes acid stain; B, basic stain; C, fat stain.

                                                    C. I. Number

Acid fuchsin	A	Acid Violet 19	42685
Acridine Orange	B	Basic Orange 14	46005
Alcian Blue 8 GX	A	Ingrain Blue 1	74240
Alcian Green (Gurr) 2GX	A	Ingrain Green 2	
Alcian Yellow GXS	A	Ingrain Yellow 1	
Alizarin Red S.	A	Mordant Red 3	58005
Aniline Blue (water soluble)	A	Acid Blue 22	42755
Aurinine O	B	Basic Yellow 2	41000

			C. I. Number
Azocarmine B	A	Acid Red 103	50090
Azocarmine G	A	Acid Red 101	50085
Azure A	B		52005
Azure II	B		
Azure B	B		52010
Basic Fuchsin	B	Basic Red 9	42500
Biebrich Scarlet	A	Acid Red 66	26905
Bismark Brown	B	Basic Brown	21000
Bordeau Red	A	Acid Red 17	16180
Brilliant Cresyl Blue	B		51010
Carmine (alum lake)	B	Natural Red 4	75470
Celestine Blue B	B	Mordant Blue 14	51050
Chlorazol Black E	A	Direct Black 38	30235
Congo Red	A	Direct Red 28	22120
Cresyl Violet	B		
Crystal Violet (Gentian Violet)	B	Basic Violet 3	42555
Dahlia (Methyl Violet 2B)	B		42535
Eosin Yellowish	A	Acid Red 87	45380
Eosin BA (Gurr)	A	Acid Red 91	45400
Erie Garnet B	A	Direct Red 10	22145
Ethyl Violet	B	Basic Violet 4	42600
Evan's Blue	A	Direct Blue 53	23860
Fast Fuchsin 6B (Fisher)	A	Acid Violet 6	16600
Fast Green FCF	A	Food Green 3	42053
Flaming Red (Fisher)	F	Pigment Red 4	12085
Gallamine Blue	B	Mordant Blue 45	51045
Gallocyanine	B	Mordant Blue 10	51030
Hematoxylin	B/M	Natural Black 1	75290
Indigo Carmine	A	Acid Blue 74	73015
Isamin Blue	A	Direct Blue 41	42700
Janus Green B	B	Diazin Greens; Union Green B	11050

			C. I. Number
Light Green SF			
Yellowish	A	Acid Green 5	42095
Lissamine Fast Yellow			
2G (Gurr)	A		
Luxol Fast Blue MBSN			
(DuPont)	A	Solvent Blue 38	
Malachite Green	B	Basic Green 4	42000
Martius Yellow	A	Acid Yellow 24	10315
Metanil Yellow	A	Acid Yellow 36	13065
Methyl Blue	A	Acid Blue 93	42780
Methylene Blue	B	Basic Blue 9	52015
Methyl Violet 2B	B	Basic Violet I	42535
Neutral Red	B	Basic Red 5	50040
New Fuchsin	B	Basic Violet 2	42520
Nile Blue Sulphate	B(F)	Basic Blue 12	51180
Nuclear Fast Red	B/M		
(Kernechtrot)			
Oil Red O	F	Solvent Red 27	26125
Orange G	A	Acid Orange 10	16230
Orcein	A		
Orcinol	A	Natural Red 28	1242
Phloxine B	A	Acid Red 92	45410
Picric Acid			
(Trinitrophenol)	A		10305
Poirrier Blue			
(Aniline Blue)	A	Acid Blue 22	42755
Ponceau de xylidine	A	Acid Red 26	16150
Purpurin	A		58205
Pyronin Y	B		45005
Quinoline Yellow	A	Acid Yellow B	47005
Safranin O	B	Basic Red 2	50240
Sirus Supra Blue			
FGL-CF	A	Direct Blue 106	51300
Sudan Black B	F	Solvent Black 3	26150
Sudan IV	F	Solvent Red 24	26105
Tartrazine	A	Acid Yellow 23	19140
Thioflavine T	B	Basic Yellow 1	49005
Thionin	B		52000
Toluidine Blue O	B	Basic Blue 17	52040
Trypan Blue	A	Direct Blue 14	23850
Trypan Red	A		22850

DYE HOUSES

Allied Chemical
National Aniline Division
Biological Stains Department
40 Rector Street
New York, N. Y. 10006

ESBE Laboratory Supplies
3431 Bathurst Street
Toronto, Ontario, Canada
Suppliers of GURR stains
(Edward Gurr, London, England. Michrome Stains)

Fisher Scientific Co.
52 Fadem Rd.
Springfield, N. J. 07081

Hartman-Leddon Co., Inc.
60th & Woodland Ave.
Philadelphia, Pa. 19143

Lipshaw Manufacturing Co.
7446 Central Avenue
Detroit, Mich. 48201

Matheson Coleman & Bell
East Rutherford, N. J. 07073

Roboz Surgical Instrument Co., Inc.
810-18th Street N. W.
Washington, D. C. 20006
(Chroma. Gesellschaft Schmid & Co.)

Chapter 10

DEHYDRATION, CLEARING, AND MOUNTING

Dehydration in alcohol serves a dual purpose; it removes
water and acts as a differentiator for excess dyes. When
placed in xylene, these reactions stop and the tissue becomes transparent. When mounted, the tissue and mounting
media should be as close as possible to the refractive
index of glass. A well-prepared section should appear
crisp and sharp when examined microscopically.

ROUTINE DEHYDRATION: HEMATOXYLIN AND EOSIN

Absolute alcohol	Three changes	3 to 5 minutes each
Absolute alcohol and xylene 50/50	Two changes	3 to 5 minutes
Xylene	Three changes	

Sections can be left in the last xylene until cover
glasses are applied. If white clouds appear when sections are placed in the first xylene, water has not been
completely removed, indicating that the last alcohol is
not absolute. Return the sections to fresh alcohol.
Solutions should be changed as necessary. Special stains
are best dehydrated in Coplin jars. Xylene used to remove paraffin should never be used for dehydration of
stained sections.

Classical mounting media were prepared from natural
resins such as Canada balsam or gum dammar and dried
slowly. Over a period of time they yellowed with age and
turned acid, causing basic dyes to fade. Many suitable
synthetic resins are now available: Clearmount, Diatex,
HSR, Permount, Pro-Texx, and XAM* to name a few. These
are dissolved to approximately 60% by weight in xylene.
toluene, or benzene.

An excellent review of the various mounting media,

*Clearmount, E. Gurr; Diatex, Scientific Products; HSR,
Hartman-Leddon Co.; Permount, Fisher Scientific Co.;
Pro-Texx, Scientific Products; XAM, G. Gurr.

also observes that toluene and benzene are highly volatile
solvents. Sections mounted in resins dissolved in these
solvents are prone to produce air spaces under by cover
glass; xylene less so. Barr recently assessed by spectro-
photometry the effects of sunlight on hematoxylin- and
eosin-stained sections mounted in various resinous media.[†]

COVER GLASS MOUNTING

Without damaging tissue, remove a slide from the xylene
with the aid of slide forceps. Allow to drain for a few
seconds and wipe excess xylene from the back of the slide
with a soft lint-free towel. As indicated previously, if
the slides are stacked in the staining rack with all tissue facing in the same direction, the danger of wiping sections off the slide is greatly reduced. Holding the slide
in a level position, place a small drop of mounting medium
near the edge of the section with a glass rod; the size of
the tissue can be used as a guide to determine the proper
amount. A clean cover glass, of the proper size, held by
the thumb and index finger at opposite corners, is placed
at an angle near the edge of the slide and allowed to
settle slowly over the section. This motion is controlled
by the index finger. Care must be taken not to trap air
bubbles; if bubbles appear, the cover glass can be raised
with the index finger and then slowly lowered again. The
tissue should not be allowed to dry at any time during
this procedure. We prefer 24-mm cover glasses, which
correspond to the width of a 3 x 1 in. microslide; clean-
up time is greatly reduced and presents a finished slide
with an attractive appearance. Narrow cover glasses (22
mm) allow mounting media to accumulate on four sides.
When removing excess media, the danger of disturbing the
cover glass is increased.
    An alternate method is to lay the cover glass on a
piece of filter paper, a drop of mounting medium is placed
on the edge of the cover glass. Place the microslide at
the edge of the cover glass and slowly rotate until the
section comes in contact with the mounting medium which
will spread, permitting the cover glass to be picked up
with the slide.
    Trapped air bubbles can be removed by applying gentle
pressure with a dissecting needle on the cover glass; if
bubbles persist, replace the slide in xylene and when the
cover glass is removed, remount the section.

*R.D. Lillie, Histopathologic Technic and Practical His-
  tochemistry, 3rd ed., McGraw Hill, 1965.
[†]W.T. Barr, Stain Tech., 45, 1 (1970).

Too thin a mounting medium, especially in thick sections, will cause air spaces to appear after the solvent has evaporated. This condition will also be evident if cover glasses are not perfectly flat or if extraneous material of sufficient size is trapped between the slide and cover glass.

If microscopic examination shows that the section is diffuse or has opaque areas, moisture due to inadequate dehydration is probably present. Remove the cover glass and all mounting media in xylene, return the slide first to fresh absolute alcohol and then to xylene and remount. Any bubbles, folds, foreign material, and excess mounting media in the completed slide should be considered as results of poor workmanship.

MOUNTING IN AQUEOUS MEDIA

When mounting loose sections (such as fat stains) in an aqueous medium, after the section has been mounted and excess water drained away, lay the slide in a horizontal position and place a drop of mounting medium in the center of the section. Slowly lower a cover glass in the same plane as the section onto the mounting medium, which should spread evenly to the periphery of the slide. In this way the section will remain centered and will not polarize to the edge of the slide.

Because sections are not attached to the slide, it is important that solutions such as glycerin jelly be thoroughly heated in a 60°C oven and kept fluid in a hot water bath during mounting. Otherwise, the solution will become too viscous and will not spread properly, causing folds to appear in the section. Do not attempt to remove trapped air bubbles by using pressure on the surface of the cover glass. This will cause fatty droplets to stream over the surface of the section, and soft tissue such as lung will become distended. Remove the cover glass carefully in warm water and carefully remount the section.

These conditions do not apply to sections mounted on albuminized slides, such as amyloid stains, which are also preserved in an aqueous medium.

Chapter 11

STAINING PROCEDURES

HEMATOXYLIN AND EOSIN

Fixation. Any routine fixative.

SOLUTIONS

1. Harris hematoxylin.

Hematoxylin	5 gm
Absolute ethyl alcohol	50 ml
Aluminum and potassium sulfate	
(potassium alum)	100 gm
Mercuric oxide (red)	2.5 gm
Distilled water	1000 ml

Dissolve, by heat, the hematoxylin in the alcohol and the potassium alum in the water. Mix the two solutions together and bring to a boil. Withdraw the flame, slowly and carefully add the mercuric chloride, heat gently, and allow to continue to boil for 4 to 5 minutes. Place the flask in cold water and cool quickly. Filter and add 40 ml of glacial acetic acid to improve nuclear staining. Filter each time before use. Effective for 1 to 2 months.

2. Acid alcohol.

70% alcohol	990 ml
Hydrochloric acid	10 ml

3. Putt's eosin counterstain.

Eosin Y	5 gm
Potassium dichromate	2.5 gm
Saturated aqueous picric acid	
(1 to 1.5%)	50 ml
Absolute ethyl alcohol	50 ml
Distilled water	400 ml

89

Dissolve the eosin in the absolute alcohol and the dichromate in the distilled water; combine the two solutions and add the picric acid.   Filter.

PROCEDURE

1.   Deparaffinize and hydrate sections.
2.   Remove mercury crystals if necessary.
3.   Stain in freshly filtered Harris' hematoxylin for 3 to 5 minutes.
4.   Wash in running tap water for 3 to 5 minutes.
5.   Differentiate in acid-alcohol until pink, 2 to 4 seconds.
6.   Wash in running tap water for 3 to 5 minutes.
7.   Blue in tap water plus a few drops of 28% ammonium hydroxide, 30 seconds to 1 minute. (Tap water, 200 ml plus 9 to 10 drops of 28% ammonium hydroxide.) Control with microscope. (Nuclei: bright blue. Cytoplasm should be colorless).
8.   Rinse in running tap water for 3 to 5 minutes.
9.   Counterstain in eosin solution for 1 to 2 minutes. Control with microscope. (Collagen, cytoplasm: pink).
10.   Rinse in tap water for 30 seconds to 1 minute.
11.   Differentiate and dehydrate in three changes of absolute alcohol, 1 to 2 minutes each.
12.   Place in absolute alcohol and xylene, 50:50, two changes, 2 to 3 minutes each.
13.   Clear in xylene, three changes.
14.   Mount in Permount.

Results.   Nuclei: blue. Cytoplasm: pink. Connective tissue and muscle fibers: pink. Red blood cells: yellow or orange. Calcium and ferrous iron: blue-purple.

Note.   If the hematoxylin is not sufficiently differentiated, when counterstaining, eosin will overlay any residual blue, resulting in a purplish tint. Freshly prepared hematoxylin stains rapidly, as the solution ages and becomes diluted with tap water; staining appears diffuse. It is good practice to change the solution completely rather than add fresh hematoxylin to an already weak solution.

Ref.   Putt, F.A., A.M.A. Arch. Path. 45, 72 (1948). Copyright American Medical Association.

WEIGERT'S IRON HEMATOXYLIN AND VAN GIESON

__Fixation.__ Any routine fixative.

SOLUTIONS

1. Weigert's hematoxylin

Solution A		Solution B	
Hematoxylin	1 gm	29% aqueous ferric	
95% ethyl alcohol	100 ml	chloride	4 ml
		Hydrochloric acid	1 ml
		Distilled water	95 ml

    Mix equal parts of solutions A and B immediately before use. Solution is good for 12 hours.

2. Van Gieson's picro-fuchsin.

Solution A		Solution B
Acid fuchsin	1 gm	Saturated aqueous solution
Saturated aqueous		of picric acid (about 1 to
solution of picric		1.5%)
acid	100 ml	

    To use, combine 1 ml of solution A with 10 ml of Solution B.

PROCEDURE

1. Deparaffinize and hydrate sections.
2. Remove mercury crystals if necessary.
3. Stain in Weigert's hematoxylin for 5 to 10 minutes.
4. Wash for 10 minutes in running tap water.
5. Counterstain sections individually with Van Gieson's picro-fuchsin for 1 minute, pouring solution on slide from a dropper bottle.
6. Differentiate with absolute alcohol, pouring on from a dropper bottle for 30 seconds, and place slide in first xylene (95% alcohol removes the picric acid stain).
7. Clear in two more changes of xylene.
8. Mount in Permount.

__Results.__ Nuclei: black. Cytoplasm: shades of brownish yellow: Red blood cells: bright yellow. Muscle fibers: brownish yellow. Collagen fibers: deep red. Coarse elastic fibers: yellow.

Note.   Effective stain for brain and spinal cord. The
             method produces a trichrome effect; one disad-
             vantage of this stain is that the picro-fuchsin
             fades in time.

Ref.   Van Gieson, J., N.Y. State J. Med., 50, (1889),
             57-60

HEIDENHAIN'S IRON HEMATOXYLIN

Fixation. Any routine fixative

SOLUTIONS

1.   Mordant and differentiator.

       Ferric ammonium sulfate (ferric alum)
          (purple crystals only)   2.5 gm
       Distilled water   100 ml

       Dissolve without heat.

2.   Hematoxylin solution.

       Hematoxylin   0.5 gm
       95% ethyl alcohol   10 ml
       Distilled water   90 ml

       Dissolve the hematoxylin in the alcohol and add
       water. Place in a bottle with cotton plug and allow
       to ripen for 4 to 5 weeks. For use, dilute with
       equal parts of distilled water. The solution may be
       used over and over.

3.   Counterstain.

       1% aqueous eosin Y or Van Gieson's picro-fuchsin.

       Van Gieson's picro-fuchsin.

Solution A		Solution B
Acid fuchsin	1 gm	Saturated aqueous solution
Saturated aqueous		of picric acid (about 1 to
solution of picric		1.5%)
acid	100 ml	

       To use, combine 1 ml of solution A with 10 ml of
       solution B.

PROCEDURE

1. Deparaffinize and hydrate sections.
2. Remove mercury crystals if necessary.
3. Mordant in ferric-ammonium-sulfate solution for 3 to 12 hours.
4. Wash quickly in tap water.
5. Stain for 1 to 24 hours in hematoxylin solution controlling under microscope (progressive staining).
6. Wash in running tap water for 5 minutes.
7. Differentiate in 2.5% ferric-ammonium-sulfate solution, controlling under microscope. Rinse in water before each examination.
8. Wash in running tap water for 30 to 60 minutes.
9. Counterstain in eosin Y or Van Gieson's picro-fuchsin for 1 minute. Agitate slide in Van Gieson's solution.
10. Differentiate eosin in 95% alcohol. Van Gieson in absolute alcohol 1 to 2 minutes.
11. Dehydrate in absolute alcohol, two changes, 1 to 2 minutes.
12. Clear in xylene two changes.
13. Mount in Permount.

Results. Chromatin, nucleoli, mitochondria, centrioles, and certain parts of striated muscle fibers: black. Other tissue elements: colored by the contrast stain used.

Ref. Mallory, F.B., Pathological Technique, Hafner Publishing Co., New York, 1968.

HARMOND'S FAST GREEN METHOD TO DEMONSTRATE MITOCHONDRIA

Fixation. Regaud's fixative.

3% aqueous potassium dichromate	40 ml
40% formaldehyde	10 ml
Prepare fresh. Discard after use.	

SOLUTIONS

1. Fast green FCF solution.

Fast green FCF	4 gm
Anilin	10 ml
Distilled water	90 ml

2.   Saturated aqueous picric acid (about 1 to 1.5%)

3.   Phosphomolybdic acid.

    Phosphomolybdic acid   1 gm
    Distilled water   100 ml

4.   Safranin O

    Safranin   1 gm
    50% alcohol   100 ml

PROCEDURE

1.   Deparaffinize and hydrate sections.
2.   Heat the fast green to $60^{\circ}C$ before use, remove from heat, and place slides in solution for 6 minutes.
3.   Rinse rapidly in distilled water.
4.   Place in picric acid solution for 10 minutes.
5.   Rinse in distilled water.
6.   Place in phosphomolybdic acid solution for 1 minute.
7.   Rinse in distilled water for 1 minute.
8.   Stain nuclei in Safranin solution for 3 minutes.
9.   Rinse in 70% alcohol, two changes.
10. Rinse in 95% alcohol, two changes.
11. Dehydrate in absolute alcohol, two changes, 1 to 2 minutes.
12. Clear in xylene, two changes.
13. Mount in Permount.

Results.   Nuclei: red. Nucleoli, erythrocytes, and plasmasomes: green. Mitochrondia: bluish green.

Ref.   Harmond, J. W. Stain Tech., 25, (1950), 69-72. Copyright the Williams and Wilkins Co.

MALLORY'S PHOSPHOTUNGSTIC ACID HEMATOXYLIN

Fixation.   Helly's fluid (mordant formalin-fixed material).

SOLUTIONS

1.   0.25% aqueous potassium permanganate.

    Potassium permanganate   0.25 gm
    Distilled water   100 ml

2.   5% aqueous oxalic acid.

    Oxalic acid   5 gm
    Distilled water   100 ml

3.   Mallory's phosphotungstic acid hematoxylin.

    Hematoxylin   1 gm
    Phosphotungstic acid   20 gm
    Distilled water   1000 ml

    Dissolve the solid ingredients in separate portions
    of water. Dissolve the hematoxylin with the aid of
    heat. When cool, combine; no preservative is neces-
    sary. Spontaneous ripening requires several weeks
    but can be accomplished at once by the addition of
    0.177 gm of potassium permanganate.

PROCEDURE

1.   Deparaffinize and hydrate sections.
2.   Remove mercury crystals.
3.   Wash in tap water.
4.   Place in potassium permanganate solution for 5
      minutes.
5.   Wash in tap water.
6.   Place in oxalic acid solution for 5 minutes.
7.   Wash in tap water.
8.   Stain in phosphotungstic acid hematoxylin for 12 to
      24 hours (overnight) in covered Coplin jar or 1 to
      2 hours at 60°C.
9.   Rinse rapidly in 95% alcohol to remove excess stain.
10.   Dehydrate rapidly in absolute alcohol, two changes,
      1 minute.
11.   Clear in xylene, two changes.
12.   Mount in Permount.

Results.   Nuclei, mitochondria, fibroglia, myoglia, and
           neuroglia fibrils, fibrin, and the contractile
           elements of striated muscle are stained blue.
           Collagen, reticulin, and the ground substance
           of cartilage and bone stain varying shades of
           yellowish to brownish red. Coarse elastic
           fibers are sometimes colored a purplish tint.

Formalin-fixed material may be mordanted in saturated
aqueous mercuric chloride for 3 hours at 58°C. Remove
mercury as above before staining. Peers, J. H., Arch.
Path., 32, 1941, pp. 446-449.

Note.   If staining tissue other than the central ner-
          vous system, omit the "Mallory Bleach" steps
          4 to 6.

Ref.   Mallory, F.B., Pathological Technique, Hafner
              Publishing Co., New York, 1968.

METHYL-GREEN-PYRONIN-METHOD

Fixation.   Carnoy's preferred. Alcohol, formalin, and
              acetic acid formalin may also be used. 10%
              formalin and Zenker's fluid unsuitable.

SOLUTIONS

1.   Methyl green-pyronin.*

PROCEDURE

1.   Deparaffinize and hydrate sections.
2.   Stain in methyl green-pyronin for 20 minutes.
3.   Rinse in cold, freshly boiled, distilled water (re-
      moves methyl green).
4.   Dehydrate in fresh acetone (removes pyronin).
5.   Clear in acetone-xylene, 50:50.
6.   Clear in xylene, two changes.
7.   Mount in Permount.

Results.   Nuclei: blue-green. Bacteria and basophil
              cytoplasm: red.

Ref.   Lillie, R.D., Histopathologic Technic and
              Practical HistoChemistry, used with permission
              of McGraw-Hill, New York, 1965.

THE FEULGEN REACTION TO DEMONSTRATE THYMONUCLEIC ACID (DNA)

Fixation.   Helly's fluid, 10% formalin. (See note for
              acid hydrolysis.)

SOLUTIONS

1.   Normal hydrochloric acid.

      Hydrochloric acid, (sp. gr. 1.19)   83.5 ml
      Distilled water   916.5 ml

2.   Schiff reagent: Bring 200 ml of distilled water to a
      boil, remove from flame, add 1 gm of basic fuchsin,

*Methyl green-pyronin (SAATHOF prepared solution), Hart-
man Leddon Co., Philadelphia, Pa. 19143

and stir until dissolved. Cool to 50°C. Filter and
add 20 ml of normal hydrochloric acid. Cool further
to 25°C. Add 1 gm of sodium or potassium metabisulfite ($Na_2S_2O_5$, $K_2S_2O_5$). Place in a dark area in a
stoppered bottle for 18 to 24 hours; solution takes
on an orange color. Add 0.5 gm of activated charcoal and shake well, then filter through a coarse
filter paper. Refrigerate in a brown stoppered
bottle of the same volume. Solution is stable for
several weeks. Use at room temperature.

3.   Sulfurous acid rinse (prepare fresh).

10% sodium metabisulfite	6 ml
Normal hydrochloric acid	5 ml
Distilled water	100 ml

4.   Counterstain.

Fast green FCF	0.5 gm
95% alcohol	100 ml

PROCEDURE

1.   Deparaffinize and hydrate sections.
2.   Remove mercury crystals if necessary.
3.   Rinse in distilled water.
4.   Rinse in normal hydrochloric acid at room tempera-
      ture for 1 minute.
5.   Place in preheated normal hydrochloric acid at 60°C
      for 4 to 5 minutes or at 50°C for 20 minutes.
6.   Rinse in distilled water.
7.   Immerse in Schiff reagent for 1 hour.
8.   Place directly in freshly prepared sulfurous acid
      rinse, three changes of 2 minutes each in closed
      Coplin jars. Discard solution.
9.   Wash in running tap water for 1 minute.
10.   Counterstain in fast green FCF for 30 seconds; if
      stain is too intense rinse in tap water.
11.   Dehydrate in 95% alcohol, then absolute alcohol, two
      changes, 1 to 2 minutes each.
12.   Clear in xylene, two changes.
13.   Mount in Permount.

<u>Results</u>. DNA is colored in shades of reddish purple.
          Background: blue-green.

Note.   Lymph node is good control material. For histo-
             chemical determinations, run a second slide
             through the procedure omitting the acid hydroly-
             sis at step 5. Time required for acid hydroly-
             sis (step 5) after various fixatives, expressed
             in minutes at 60°C:

             Bouin-Allen   22   Helly   8
             Carnoy   8   Petrunkevitch   3
             Carnoy-LeBrun   6   Regaud   14
             Champy   25   Susa   18
             Zenker   5   Bouin is not recommended

Ref.   Pearse, A. G. E., Histochemistry Theoretical and
             Applied, Little, Brown, Boston, 1960.

MASSON'S TRICHROME STAIN FOR CONNECTIVE TISSUE (MODIFIED)

Fixation. Helly's fluid or 10% formalin.

SOLUTIONS

1.   Saturated picric acid (9%) in absolute alcohol.

2.   Lendrum's celestin blue. Dissolve 5 gm of iron alum
      (ferric ammonium sulfate) at room temperature in 100
      ml of distilled water. Bring to a boil, add 0.5 gm
      of celestin blue, and boil for 3 minutes. Filter
      when cool and add 14 ml of glycerin. Solution lasts
      for about 1 month. Filter before use.

3.   Mayer's haemalum.

      Hematoxylin crystals   1 gm
      Sodium iodate   0.2 gm
      Aluminum and ammonium sulfate
         (ammonia alum)   50 gm
      Distilled water   1000 ml
      Chloral hydrate   50 gm
      Citric acid   1 gm

      Dissolve hematoxylin, sodium iodate and the ammonia
      alum overnight in 1000 ml of distilled water; add
      the chloral hydrate and citric acid. Boil for 5
      minutes; when cool, it is ready for use. The solu-
      tion keeps well.

4.   Acid alcohol. 1 ml of hydrochloric acid in 99 ml of
      70% alcohol.

5.   Acid fuchsin solution.

      Acid fuchsin   0.6 gm
      Ponceau de xylidine   1.4 gm
      Distilled water   400 ml
      Glacial acetic acid   2 ml

6.   Phosphomolybdic acid   1 gm
      Distilled water   100 ml

7.   Light green solution.

      Light green SF yellowish   2 gm
      Distilled water   99 ml
      Glacial acetic acid   1 ml

8.   Aniline blue solution (alternate counterstain)

      Aniline blue   2.5 gm
      Distilled water   98 ml
      Glacial acetic acid   2 ml

9.   1% aqueous glacial acetic acid.

PROCEDURE

 1.   Deparaffinize and hydrate sections.
 2.   Remove mercury crystals if necessary.
 3.   Mordant formalin-fixed tissue in alcoholic picric
      acid for 10 minutes.
 4.   Wash well in running tap water.
 5.   Rinse in distilled water.
 6.   Stain in Lendrum's celestin blue for 10 minutes.
 7.   Wash in tap water.
 8.   Stain in Mayer's haemalum for 5 minutes.
 9.   Wash well in tap water. Check nuclei under micro-
      scope; if too dark, differentiate in acid alcohol
      for a few seconds.
10.   Wash well in running tap water.
11.   Stain in acid fuchsin solution for 5 minutes.
12.   Rinse in distilled water.
13.   Differentiate in phosphomolybdic acid solution for 5
      minutes. (Control with microscope.)
14.   Without rinsing, counterstain in light green solu-
      tion for 1 minute or anilin blue for 2 to 5 minutes.
      (We prefer the light green counterstain.)
15.   Rinse in distilled water.
16.   Differentiate in phosphomolybdic acid solution for
      5 minutes, discard. (Check with microscope.) Omit
      this step with anilin blue.

17.   Place in 1% acetic acid solution for 3 to 5 minutes;
       discard solution.
18.   Dehydrate in 95% alcohol, then absolute alcohol, two
       changes, 1 to 2 minutes each.
19.   Clear in xylene, two changes.
20.   Mount in Permount.

Results.   Nuclei: black. Cytoplasm and muscle fibers:
            red. Collagen: blue or green depending on the
            counterstain.

Note.   The double nuclear staining procedure as out-
            lined by Lendrum eliminates loss of nuclear de-
            tail by acid solutions.

Ref.   Lendrum, A.C., Celestin blue as a nuclear
            stain, J. Path. Bact., 40, (1935), 415-416.
            Masson, P., personal communication.

MALLORY'S PHLOXINE-METHYLENE BLUE STAIN

Fixation.   Zenker's or Helly's fluid. 10% formalin may
             also be used.

SOLUTIONS

1.   Phloxine B.

      Phloxine B   2.5 gm
      Distilled water   100 ml

2.   Methylene blue-azure II.

      Methylene blue   1 gm   Azure II   1 gm
      Borax (sodium borate) 1 gm   Distilled water 100 ml
      Distilled water   100 ml

      Working solution. Take 5 ml of methylene blue and
      5 ml of azure II. Add 90 ml of distilled water;
      this solution should be mixed fresh each time and
      filtered.

3.   Differentiating solution. 100 ml of 95% alcohol to
      which has been added 2 to 5 ml of a 10% solution of
      Colophonium (rosin white lumps) dissolved in abso-
      lute alcohol or in Putt's solution; absolute alco-
      hol 50 ml, glacial acetic acid 4 to 5 drops.

PROCEDURE

1. Deparaffinize and hydrate sections.
2. Remove mercury crystals if necessary.
3. Stain in phloxine solution for 1 hour or longer in
    60°C oven, in covered Coplin jar.
4. Allow solution to cool before pouring it off and
    rinse sections carefully in distilled water. The
    solution may be used over and over.
5. Place in methylene blue-azure II solution for 5 to
    10 minutes. Agitate the slides gently to ensure an
    even staining.
6. Transfer to distilled water and differentiate indi-
    vidually in rosin solution. Keep slides in constant
    back-and-forth motion to ensure even differentiation
    until the background becomes pink and the nuclei re-
    main blue (control with microscope).
7. Dehydrate rapidly in three changes of absolute alco-
    hol, 1 minute each. (All rosin must be removed.)
8. Clear in xylene, two changes.
9. Mount in Permount.

Results.   Nuclei and bacteria: blue. Plasma cell cyto-
           plasm: blue. Mucin: blue. Connective tissue:
           bright rose. After Zenker fixation hyaline
           stains intensely red.

Note.   It is important to get a deep stain with phlox-
           ine because the methylene blue dissolves it or
           washes it out to a considerable extent. The
           phloxine must be used first because the methy-
           lene blue is readily soluble in an aqueous solu-
           tion of phloxine and therefore is quickly ex-
           tracted if the phloxine is used after it, while,
           on the other hand, phloxine is only slightly
           soluble in an aqueous solution of methylene blue.

Ref.   Mallory, F. B., Pathological Technique, Hafner
           Publishing Co., New York, 1968.

THOMAS' PHLOXINE-METHYLENE BLUE METHOD.

Fixation.   10% formalin, Helly's fluid.

SOLUTIONS

1.   Phloxine solution.

     Phloxine B   0.5 gm

Distilled water	100 ml
Glacial acetic acid	0.2 ml

Filter before use.

2. Azure B-methylene blue solution.

Methylene blue	0.25 gm
Azure B (C.I. No. 52010)	0.25 gm
Borax (sodium borate)	0.25 gm
Distilled water	100 ml

3.   0.2% aqueous acetic acid.

PROCEDURE

1.   Deparaffinize and hydrate sections.
2.   Remove mercury crystals if necessary.
3.   Stain in phloxine solution for 1 to 2 minutes.
4.   Rinse well in distilled water.
5.   Stain in methylene blue solution 1/2 to 1 minute.
6.   Partially destain in 0.2% acetic acid.
7.   Continue differentiation in 95% alcohol, three
     changes. (Control with microscope.)
8.   Dehydrate in absolute alcohol, two changes, 1 to 2
     minutes each.
9.   Clear in xylene, two changes.
10. Mount in Permount.

Results.   Nuclei: blue. Plasma cell cytoplasm: blue.
           Other tissue elements: rose to red.

Ref.   Thomas, J.T., Stain Tech., 28 (1953), 311-312.
           Copyright The Williams and Wilkins Co.

MAXIMOW'S HEMATOXYLIN-AZURE II-EOSIN METHOD

Fixation. 10% formalin, Helly's or Zenker's fluids.

SOLUTIONS

1.   Mayer's haemalum.

Hematoxylin crystals	1 gm
Sodium iodate	0.2 gm
Aluminum and ammonium sulfate	
(ammonia alum)	50 gm
Distilled water	1000 ml
Chloral hydrate	50 gm
Citric acid	1 gm

Dissolve hematoxylin, sodium iodate and the ammonia alum overnight in 1000 ml of distilled water; add the chloral hydrate and citric acid. Boil for 5 minutes; when cool, it is ready for use. The solution keeps well.

2.   Azure II. Eosin-Y solution (stock).

1:1000 aqueous eosin-Y
1:1000 aqueous azure II

Working solution
1:1000 eosin-Y   5 ml
Fresh distilled water   40 ml
1:1000 azure II   5 ml

Mix in the order above and discard after use.

PROCEDURE

1.   Deparaffinize and hydrate sections.
2.   Remove mercury crystals if necessary.
3.   Stain in Mayer's haemalum for 5 minutes. This may be omitted if a less dense nuclear stain is desired.
4.   Wash in running tap water.
5.   Rinse in distilled water.
6.   Stain in azure II-Eosin-Y solution for 18 to 24 hours.
7.   Differentiate sections individually in 95% alcohol until the gross blue clouds cease to come out in the alcohol, and the red cells and collagen are pink. (Control with microscope.)
8.   Dehydrate in absolute alcohol, two changes, 1 minute each.
9.   Clear in xylene, two changes.
10.   Mount in Permount.

Results.   Nuclei: blue. Basophil. leukocytes, and mast cell granules: purple to violet. Red blook corpuscles: pink. Cytoplasm: blue to pink. Secretion granules and eosinophil granules: pink.

Ref.   Mallory, F.B. Pathological Technique, Hafner Publishing Co., New York, 1968.

HEIDENHAIN'S AZAN-CARMINE ANILINE BLUE METHOD

Fixation. Zenker's or Helly's fluid.

SOLUTIONS

1. Azocarmine B or G   1 gm
    Distilled water   100 ml
    Glacial acetic acid   1 ml

    Azocarmine B is more readily soluble in water; azo-
    carmine G is preferred. If azocarmine G is used,
    add 1 gm to the 100 ml of water, bring it to a boil,
    cool to room temperature, and filter through a coarse
    filter paper in the paraffin oven at 60°C, so that
    the fine particles of dye will also pass through.
    After cooling, add 1 ml of glacial acetic acid.

2. Alcohol-aniline oil solution (McGregor).

    Aniline oil   1 ml
    95% alcohol   100 ml

    Shake well.

3. 1% glacial acetic acid solution.

    95% alcohol   99 ml
    Acetic acid   1 ml

4. Phosphotungstic acid solution.

    Phosphotungstic acid   5 gm
    Distilled water   100 ml

5. Aniline blue-Orange-G solution.

    Aniline blue   0.5 gm
    Orange G   2 gm
    Distilled water   100 ml
    Glacial acetic acid   8 ml

PROCEDURE

1. Deparaffinize and hydrate sections.
2. Remove mercury crystals.
3. Stain in the azocarmine solution for 1 hour at 60°C
    in covered Coplin jar.
4. Allow to cool to room temperature; wash in tap water.
5. Differentiate in aniline oil-alcohol solution, 1 to 3
    minutes, until nuclei are red. (Check with micro-
    scope.)
6. Rinse in acetic acid alcohol.

7. Mordant in phosphotungstic acid solution for 2 hours.
8. Wash in distilled water.
9. Stain in aniline blue-Orange G solution for 1 to 2 hours.
10. Wash quickly in distilled water.
11. Differentiate in absolute alcohol, two changes. (Control with microscope.)
12. Clear in xylene, two changes.
13. Mount in Permount.

Results.   Collagen and reticulin: deep blue. Chromatin: red. Nuclei: orange red. Cytoplasm: pink Mucin: blue. Fibrin: red.

DAVIDOFF MODIFICATION FOR FORMALIN-FIXED TISSUES

Paraffin Sections of Formalin-Fixed Tissue

1. Deparaffinize and hydrate sections.
2. Place for 1 hour in dilute ammonium hydroxide (10 ml of ammonium hydroxide 28% to 100 ml of distilled water).
3. Wash for 1 hour in running tap water.
4. Place in Helly's or Zenker's fluid for 1 hour.
5. Wash for 1 hour in running tap water.
6. Remove mercury crystals and stain as usual.

Blocks of Formalin-Fixed Tissue

1. Leave blocks in ammonia water as above for 2 days in 40°C oven.
2. Wash for 24 hours in running tap water.
3. Place blocks in Zenker's fluid for 12 hours or in Helly's fluid for 5 hours.
4. Wash for 12 hours in running tap water.
5. Embed in paraffin, remove mercury crystals, and stain as usual.

Ref.   Mallory, F. B., Pathological Technique, Hafner Publishing Co., N. Y. 1968. McGregor, S., Am. J. Path., 5 (1929), 545-557. Davidoff, L. M., Am. J. Path., 4 (1928), 493.

SCHMORL'S METHOD TO DEMONSTRATE COMPACT BONE

Fixation.   10% formalin.

SOLUTIONS

1.   Thionin solution.

    Thionin, 0.25% in 50% alcohol   2 ml
    Distilled water   10 ml

2.   Saturated aqueous phosphotungstic acid.

    160 gm to 64 ml water

3.   Picric acid   0.5 gm
    Distilled water   100 ml

4.   Formalin solution.

    Formaldehyde 40%   20 ml
    Distilled water   20 ml

PROCEDURE

1.   Decalcify bone.
2.   Embed in paraffin.
3.   Cut sections at 5 microns.
4.   Deparaffinize and hydrate sections.
5.   Stain for 5 minutes in thionin solution.
6.   Rinse in water.
7.   Differentiate for 1 to 2 minutes in 95% alcohol.
8.   Rinse in water.
9.   Differentiate in phosphotungstic acid solution for
     1 to 5 minutes or in picric acid solution for 30 to
     60 seconds. (Control with microscope.)
10. Wash in running tap water for 10 minutes.
11. Fix color in formalin solution for 1 to 2 hours.
12. Dehydrate in 95% alcohol and then absolute alcohol,
     two changes, 1 to 2 minutes each.
13. Clear in xylene, two changes.
14. Mount in Permount.

Results. Cytoplasm of bone cells, their processes, and
          the lacunae in which the cells rest are blue to
          black. Bone matrix is light blue with phospho-
          tungstic acid or yellow with picric acid.

Ref.   McManus, J. F. A. and Mowry, R. W., Staining
          Methods Histologic and Histochemical, Hoeber
          Medical Division, Harper & Row, New York, 1963.

LAIDLAW'S LITHIUM SILVER CARBONATE METHOD TO
DEMONSTRATE RETICULIN

Fixation. 10% formalin or Bouin's fluid. Helly's or
          Zenker's fluids may be used; however, the stain-
          ing then is not as delicate, since the silver
          deposits appear granular, probably due to the
          presence of mercury.

SOLUTIONS

1.   Potassium permanganate   0.25 gm
     Distilled water   100 ml

2.   Oxalic acid   5 gm
     Distilled water   100 ml

3.   Modified Hortega's lithium silver carbonate. In a
     chemically clean, glass-stoppered, 1000-ml graduate
     make up 100 ml of 20% aqueous nitrate (20 gm per 100
     ml of distilled water). To this solution add 400 ml
     of a saturated aqueous solution of lithium carbonate
     (6 gm per 500 ml of water). This solution should be
     prepared fresh; a yellowish white precipitate will
     form. Wash the precipitate 6 to 7 times with fresh
     distilled water, allowing it to settle between each
     washing. Decant carefully so as not to loose the
     precipitate. Dissolve the remaining precipitate
     with fresh 28% ammonium hydroxide from a dropper
     bottle, adding 2 to 3 drops at a time, shaking the
     graduate continually until only a few granules re-
     main; do not add ammonia to excess. The solution is
     then made up to 200 ml with distilled water and fil-
     tered through a Whatman No. 1 filter paper into a
     chemically clean, brown, glass-stoppered bottle.
     The solution will keep for many months and may be
     used repeatedly. Filter before and after use.

4.   Reducer.

     40% formaldehyde   1 ml
     Distilled water   99 ml

5.   Toning solution: 1:500 yellow gold chloride. Yellow
     gold chloride may be prepared as follows. Wash the
     label off a 15-grain vial of Merck yellow gold chlo-
     ride in hot water. Rinse well in distilled water,
     place the vial in a 500-ml glass-stoppered, chemical-
     ly clean, brown bottle. Replace the stopper, sharply

shake the bottle to break vial, and add 500 ml of
distilled water.

6.   Sodium thiosulfate (hypo)   5 gm
      Distilled water   100 ml

PROCEDURE

1.   Cut sections at 5 microns and mount on slides with
      the Masson gelatin method. Egg albumin may be used
      if the slides are left overnight in the 50°C oven.
      Coating these slides with a thin (0.5%) solution of
      celloidin during dehydration after absolute alcohol
      will prevent the loss of sections during staining.
2.   Remove mercury crystals if necessary.
3.   Oxidize all sections in potassium permanganate for
      5 minutes.
4.   Wash well in running tap water.
5.   Reduce in 5% oxalic acid for 5 minutes.
6.   Wash well in tap water.
7.   Rinse in three changes of distilled water 2 to 3
      minutes each.
8.   Place in lithium silver solution which has been pre-
      viously filtered and heated in the oven to 50°C in
      covered Coplin jar. The sections are left in the
      silver until they take on a light brown color, about
      15 minutes to 1/2 hour. Zenker- or Helly- fixed
      materials stain more rapidly than formalin and
      should be stained separately.
9.   Rinse in two changes of distilled water.
10.   Reduce in 1% solution of formalin, two changes of
      1 to 2 minutes each. Discard the first change al-
      most immediately and allow sections to reduce in
      second change for balance of time. Discard form-
      alin.
11.   Rinse in distilled water.
12.   Tone in 1:500 yellow gold chloride for 10 minutes.
      (Discard.)
13.   Rinse in distilled water 2 to 3 minutes.
14.   Check sections under microscope; if collagen does
      not have a reddish purple tinge, place in 5% oxalic
      acid for 5 minutes.
15.   Wash in tap water for 5 minutes.
16.   Fix in 5% sodium thiosulfate for 5 minutes.
17.   Wash in tap water for 5 minutes.
18.   Dehydrate in 95% alcohol, then absolute alcohol,
      two changes, 1 to 2 minutes each.
19.   Clear in xylene, two changes.
20.   Mount in Permount.

Results.   Collagen fibers: reddish purple; the more
            delicate reticulin fibers appear as fine black
            threads. After Bouin's fluid the cytoplasm of
            the epithelial cells is colored black and the
            nuclei are colorless. After formalin fixation,
            the nuclei are black and the cytoplasm color-
            less.

Note.   The demonstration of reticulin in this tech-
            nique is due to a deposit of lithium silver
            carbonate upon the fibers. Care must be exer-
            cised to avoid all extraneous precipitates.
            All glassware used for preparing solutions and
            for staining must be chemically clean and
            rinsed in glass-distilled water. If the silver
            solution is properly prepared, consistent
            staining for many months is possible. This is
            our preferred method.

Ref.   Laidlaw, G.F., Amer. J. Path., 5, (1929)
            239-247.

GRIDLEY'S METHOD TO DEMONSTRATE RETICULIN

Fixation.   10% formalin, Helly's fluid.

SOLUTIONS

1.   Periodic acid.

      Periodic acid   0.5 gm
      Distilled water   100 ml

2.   Silver nitrate.

      Silver nitrate   2 gm
      Distilled water   100 ml

3.   Diammine silver hydroxide solution. To 20 ml of 5%
      aqueous silver nitrate solution in an acid- clean
      graduate cylinder add 20 drops of a 10% aqueous
      sodium hydroxide solution. Then add from a dropper
      bottle, drop by drop, fresh 28% ammonium hydroxide
      until only a few granules remain in the cylinder.
      Bring the volume up to 60 ml with distilled water,
      filter, and use at once. Prepare fresh each time.

4. Reducing solution.

    Formaldehyde 40%   30 ml
    Distilled water   70 ml

5. Toning solution.

    1:500 yellow gold chloride

6. Sodium thiosulfate (hypo)

    Sodium thiosulfate   5 gm
    Distilled water   100 ml

7. Nuclear fast red (Kernechtrot) counterstain. Dis-
    solve 0.1 gm nuclear fast red in 100 ml of a 5%
    aqueous aluminum sulfate solution with the aid of
    heat. Cool and filter. Add a crystal of thymol as
    a preservative. The solution keeps well at room
    temperature and can be reused.

PROCEDURE

1.   Deparaffinize and hydrate sections.
2.   Remove mercury crystals if necessary.
3.   Place in periodic acid for 15 minutes.
4.   Rinse in distilled water.
5.   Place in 2% silver nitrate solution for 30 minutes.
6.   Rinse in distilled water.
7.   Place in Diammine silver solution for 15 minutes in
     covered Coplin jar.
8.   Rinse very quickly in distilled water.
9.   Reduce in formalin solution for 3 minutes. (Discard.)
10. Rinse in several changes of distilled water.
11. Tone in gold chloride solution for 5 to 10 minutes.
     (Discard.)
12. Wash in distilled water.
13. Fix in 5% sodium thiosulfate solution for 5 minutes.
14. Wash for 5 to 10 minutes in tap water.
15. Counterstain in nuclear fast red for 10 minutes.
16. Rinse in tap water.
17. Dehydrate in 95% alcohol then absolute alcohol, two
     changes, 1 to 2 minutes each.
18. Clear in xylene, two changes.
19. Mount in Permount.

Results. Reticulin fibers: black. Nuclei: red.

Note.   All glassware should be chemically clean and
          rinsed in distilled water.

Ref.   Gridley, M.F., Amer. J. Clin. Path., 21,
                  (1951), 879-881.

GOMORI'S MODIFICATION OF THE BIELSCHOWSKI-MARESCH
METHOD FOR RETICULIN

Fixation.   Practically all of the usual fixatives in-
             cluding alcohol may be used. After fixation
             in Bouin's fluid, however, the cytoplasm may
             stain undesirably heavily.

SOLUTIONS

1.   Oxidizer. Acidified potassium permanganate.

      Potassium permanganate   5 gm
      Distilled water   500 ml
      Concentrated sulfuric acid   2.5 ml

2.   Decolorizer.

      Potassium metabisulfite   2 gm
      Distilled water   100 ml

3.   Sensitizer.

      Ferric ammonium sulfate (iron alum)   2 gm
      Distilled water   100 ml

4.   Diammine silver hydroxide solution. In a chemically
      clean glass vessel, place 40 ml of a 10% solution of
      silver nitrate. Add 10 ml of a 40% aqueous solution
      of potassium hydroxide. Add 28% ammonium hydroxide,
      drop by drop, while shaking the container continu-
      ously, until the precipitate is completely dissolved.
      Again add, cautiously, 10% silver nitrate solution
      drop by drop, until the resulting precipitate easily
      disappears on shaking the solution. Make up the
      solution to twice its volume with distilled water,
      then filter. Solution will keep in a brown stop-
      pered bottle for 2 days. Filter before use.

5.   Reducing solution.

      Formaldehyde 40%   20 ml
      Distilled water   80 ml

6.   Toning solution.

      1:500 yellow gold chloride

7.   Reducer.

      Potassium metabisulfite   2 gm
      Distilled water   100 ml

8.   Sodium thiosulfate (hypo)   2 gm
      Distilled water   100 ml

PROCEDURE

1.   Deparaffinize and hydrate sections.
2.   Remove mercury crystals if necessary.
3.   Oxidize sections in acidified potassium permanganate
      for 1 to 2 minutes.
4.   Rinse in distilled water.
5.   Decolorize in potassium metabisulfite for 1 minute.
6.   Wash in tap water for several minutes. After this
      step the sections should have a pale pink color.
      If there is the slightest brown staining, repeat
      steps 3 and 5 until the desired pink color to the
      sections is obtained. This may require repeating
      the steps once or twice. (Control under micro-
      scope.)
7.   Sensitize in ferric ammonium sulfate for 1 minute.
8.   Wash in tap water for 3 to 5 minutes.
9.   Wash well in two changes of distilled water.
10.   Place in Diammine silver hydroxide solution for 1
      minute.
11.   Rinse quickly in distilled water for 1 to 5 seconds.
12.   Reduce in formalin solution for 3 to 5 minutes.
      (Discard.)
13.   Wash well in distilled water for a few minutes.
14.   Tone in yellow gold chloride for 10 minutes.
      (Discard.)
15.   Rinse in distilled water.
16.   Reduce in potassium metabisulfite for 1 minute.
17.   Fix in sodium thiosulfate for 1 to 2 minutes.
18.   Wash in tap water for 5 minutes.
19.   Counterstain if desired in hematoxylin or Van Gie-
      son's counterstain.
20.   Dehydrate in 95% alcohol, Van Gieson in absolute
      alcohol.
21.   Dehydrate in absolute alcohol, two changes, 1 to 2
      minutes each.
22.   Clear in xylene, two changes.
23.   Mount in Permount.

Results.   Fine fibers of reticulin or collagen: black.
              In sections that have not been counterstained,
              the larger bundles of collagen will vary in
              color from pink to brown. Nuclei and cyto-
              plasm will appear in varying shades of gray.

Note.   All glassware should be chemically clean and
              rinsed in distilled water.

Ref.   Gomori, G., Amer. J. Path., 13, (1937) 993-1001.

HUMASON AND LUSHBAUGH METHOD TO DEMONSTRATE
RETICULIN, COLLAGEN, AND ELASTIN

Fixation. Any routine fixative.

SOLUTIONS

1.   Silver nitrate   2 gm
     Distilled water   100 ml

2.   Diammine silver hydroxide solution.

     Silver nitrate   5 gm
     Distilled water   100 ml

     Sodium hydroxide   10 gm
     Distilled water   100 ml

     To 20 ml of silver nitrate, add 20 drops of 10% so-
     dium hydroxide; a precipitate forms. With constant
     shaking add 28% ammonium hydroxide drop by drop from
     a dropper bottle until a few grains of precipitate
     remain undissolved; do not add ammonia to excess.
     Add distilled water to bring the volume up to 60 ml.
     Filter. Use at once. Discard after use.

3.   Reducing solution.

     Formaldehyde 40%   30 ml
     Distilled water   100 ml

4.   Toning solution.

     1:500 yellow gold chloride.

5.   Sodium thiosulfate   5 gm
     Distilled water   100 ml

6.   Orcein solution.

      Orcein   0.5 gm
      70% ethyl alcohol   100 ml
      Concentrated hydrochloric acid   0.6-1.0 ml

7.   Phosphomolybdic acid   1 gm
      Distilled water   100 ml

8.   Sirus blue*   2 gm
      Distilled water   100 ml
      Glacial acetic acid   2 ml

PROCEDURE

1.   Deparaffinize and hydrate sections.
2.   Remove mercury crystals if necessary.
3.   Rinse well in distilled water.
4.   Transfer to 2% silver nitrate for 30 minutes.
5.   Rinse in distilled water for 2 to 3 seconds.
6.   Place in Diammine silver hydroxide for 15 minutes.
7.   Rinse quickly in two changes of distilled water.
8.   Reduce in 30% formalin for 3 minutes, agitate
      slightly. (Discard.)
9.   Rinse in distilled water.
10.   Tone in yellow gold chloride for 5 to 10 minutes.
      (Discard.)
11.   Rinse in distilled water.
12.   Fix in 5% sodium thiosulfate for 5 minutes.
13.   Rinse in 70% alcohol.
14.   Stain in orcein solution at 37°C for 15 minutes.
15.   Rinse in 70% alcohol, then in distilled water.
16.   Transfer to 5% phosphomolybdic acid for 5 minutes.
17.   Rinse in three changes of distilled water, 10 sec-
      onds each.
18.   Stain in Sirus blue for 5 minutes.
19.   Wash in 2 to 3 changes of distilled water, 10 sec-
      onds each.
20.   Dehydrate in 3 changes of absolute alcohol, 2 to 3
      minutes.
21.   Clear in xylene, two changes.
22.   Mount in Permount.

Results.   Reticulin: black. Elastin: red. Collagen:
           blue.

*Sirus supre blue FGL-CF (Direct blue 106, C. I. No.
 51300), Roboz Surgical Instrument Co., Washington, D. C.
 20006.

Note.   All glassware whould be chemically clean. Do
             not use metallic forceps in silver solutions.

Ref.   Humason, D.L. and Lushbaugh, C. C. Stain Tech.,
             44, 2 (1969), 105-106. Copyright the William
             and Witkins Co., Personal Communication (Sirus
             Supre Blue)

SLIDDERS, FRAZER, AND LENDRUM'S METHOD TO
DEMONSTRATE RETICULIN

Fixation. Formol-sublimate, 10% formalin.

SOLUTIONS

1.   Phosphotungstic acid   30 gm
     Distilled water   100 ml

2.   Sensitizer.

     Tannic acid   1 gm
     Glacial acetic acid   2 ml
     95% alcohol   100 ml

3.   Diargentine silver carbonate. Pipette 5 ml of 10%
     aqueous silver nitrate followed by 5 ml of a satu-
     rated aqueous lithium carbonate (approx. 2 gm per
     100 ml) into a 250 ml chemically clean flask. Mix
     thoroughly. Wash the precipitate by adding 50 ml of
     distilled water and agitating. Allow the precipi-
     tate to settle and carefully decant the supernate;
     repeat this washing twice. Suspend the precipitate
     in 10 ml of distilled water and dissolve by adding
     dilute ammonium hydroxide (28% ammonium hydroxide
     diluted with 2 parts of distilled water) drop by
     drop with constant agitation. Use absolutely no
     more ammonia than what will just dissolve the pre-
     cipitate. Leave the solution uncovered for several
     hours to allow traces of free ammonia to escape.
     Pipette in 10 ml of 10% aqueous silver nitrate and
     mix thoroughly. Wash, suspend, and dissolve the re-
     sulting precipitate as before. Avoid excess ammonia.
     Allow a little of the precipitate to remain undis-
     solved. Make up to 50 ml with distilled water and
     allow to stand for 24 hours before use. Store in a
     glass-stoppered brown bottle. Solution lasts for
     months.

4. Reducer.

40% formaldehyde	10 ml
Distilled water	90 ml
Diargentine silver carbonate	1 ml

An opalescence forms on the addition of the diargentine carbonate. This gradually settles as granules. Discard solution when dirty.

5.	Sodium thiosulfate	5 gm
	Distilled water	100 ml

6. Toning solution.

1:500 aqueous yellow gold chloride.

PROCEDURE

1. Deparaffinize and hydrate sections.
2. Remove mercury crystals if necessary.
3. Place in phosphotungstic acid solution for 3 minutes.
4. Wash in running tap water for 2 to 3 minutes.
5. Rinse both sides of slide with 95% alcohol.
6. Place in tannic acid solution for 2 minutes.
7. Rinse slide in distilled water.
8. Place in diargentine silver at room temperature for 5 to 7 minutes in covered Coplin jar.
9. Rinse both sides of slide well with distilled water.
10. Place in reducing solution for 30 seconds. (Discard.)
11. Wash in running tap water.
12. Place in sodium thiosulfate for 20 to 30 seconds.
13. Wash in running tap water.
14. Tone in gold chloride for 2 to 3 minutes. (Discard.)
15. Wash in running tap water.
16. Rinse quickly in sodium thiosulfate. Place immediately in running tap water. May be repeated if necessary. This cleans up background.
17. Dehydrate in 95% alcohol then absolute alcohol, two changes, 1 to 2 minutes each.
18. Clear in xylene, two changes.
19. Mount in Permount.

Results.   Reticulin and collagen fibers: black.

Ref.   Slidders, W., Frazer, D. S. and Lendrum, A. C., J. Path. Bact., 75, 2 (1958), 478-481.

NASSAR AND SHANKLIN METHOD TO DEMONSTRATE RETICULIN

Fixation. 10% formalin.

SOLUTIONS

1. Potassium permanganate   0.5 gm
    Distilled water   100 ml

2. Sulfuric acid   0.5 ml
    Distilled water   100 ml

3. Oxidizing solution.

    Equal parts of 1 and 2. Discard after use.

4. Oxalic acid   2 gm
    Distilled water   100 ml

5. Silver nitrate   2 gm
    Distilled water   100 ml
    Pyridine   30 drops

6. Lillie's Diammine-Hydroxide silver solution. Place
    1 ml of 28% ammonium hydroxide in a chemically
    clean flask and add 7 ml of 10% aqueous solution of
    silver nitrate. Continue to add 10% silver drop by
    drop, shaking between each addition, until a faint
    permanent turbidity remains after the last drop
    added. Dilute with an equal volume of distilled
    water. Solution lasts for 2 to 3 days. Filter be-
    fore use.

7. Reducer.

    40% formaldehyde   2 ml
    Distilled water   98 ml

8. Toning solution.

    1:500 aqueous yellow gold chloride

9. Sodium thiosulfate   5 gm
    Distilled water   100 ml

10. Mayer's hemalum.

    Hematoxylin crystals   1 gm
    Sodium iodate   0.2 gm

Aluminum and ammonium sulfate
  (ammonia alum)   50 gm
Distilled water   1000 ml
Chloral hydrate   50 gm
Citric acid   1 gm

Dissolve hematoxylin, sodium iodate, and the ammonia alum overnight in 1000 ml of distilled water;
add the chloral hydrate and citric acid. Boil for
5 minutes; when cool, it is ready for use. The
solution keeps well.

PROCEDURE

1. Deparaffinize and hydrate sections.
2. Rinse in distilled water.
3. Place in oxidizing solution for 1 to 2 minutes;
    sections take on a brown color.
4. Rinse in distilled water.
5. Decolorize in oxalic acid solution for 2 minutes.
6. Rinse in distilled water.
7. Pass section up through 60, 70, 80, and 95% alcohol,
    1 to 2 minutes each.
8. Place in silver-pyridine solution at 50°C for 30
    minutes to 1 hour in covered Coplin jar. Sections
    may be left at room temperature for longer periods
    of time. Finer fibers are best demonstrated by a
    shorter period of time in the silver, coarse fibers
    by the longer period with a loss of finer fibers.
9. Rinse quickly in 95% alcohol.
10. Place in Lillie's Diammine silver hydroxide solu-
    tion to which has been added 3 drops of pyridine
    per 10 ml of solution for 5 minutes at 50°C.
11. Rinse in 95% alcohol.
12. Reduce in formalin solution for 2 minutes. (Discard.)
13. Wash in distilled water.
14. Tone in gold chloride for 5 to 10 minutes or until
    sections turn gray. (Discard.)
15. Rinse in distilled water.
16. Fix in sodium thiosulfate for 5 minutes.
17. Wash in tap water.
18. If desired, stain nuclei in Mayer's hemalum, dif-
    ferentiate in acid alcohol (1 ml hydrochloric acid
    in 99 ml of 70% alcohol). Wash in tap water. Sec-
    tions may also be counterstained in Van Gieson's
    picro-fuchsin diluted to half with distilled water.
19. Dehydrate in 95% alcohol. Van Gieson in absolute
    alcohol.
20. Dehydrate in absolute alcohol, two changes, 1 to 2
    minutes each.

21.   Clear in xylene, two changes.
22.   Mount in Permount.

Results.   Reticulin: black. Collagen fibers: lavender;
           red if counterstained with Van Gieson. Nuclei:
           blue if counterstained in Mayer's hemalum.

Ref.   Nassar, T.K. and Shanklin, W.M., A.M.A.
           Arch. Path., 71, (1961), 611-614. Copy-
           right American Medical Association

VERHOEFF'S METHOD FOR ELASTIC FIBERS

Fixation. Helly's or Zenker's fluids or 10% formalin.

SOLUTIONS

1.   Verhoeff's elastic tissue solutions.

      A.   Hematoxylin   5 gm
            Absolute alcohol   100 ml

      Dissolve the hematoxylin in the alcohol with the aid
      of gentle heat (water bath). Cool and filter and
      store in a tightly stoppered bottle.

      B.   Verhoeff's iodine solution.

            Iodine crystals   2 gm
            Potassium iodide   4 gm
            Distilled water   100 ml

      Dissolve the potassium iodide in a small amount of
      distilled water. Add the iodine and shake well,
      then add the balance of the distilled water.

      C.   Ferric chloride solution.

            Ferric chloride (FeCL2)   10 gm
            Distilled water   100 ml

            Working solution. Combine in order given.

            Solution A   60 ml
            Solution B   24 ml
            Solution C   24 ml

Filter before use. The combined solution is stable
for about 24 hours. <u>Note</u>. These proportions are
taken from McClung's Microscopical Technique. Mallory and Lillie recommend the following formula:
hematoxylin 40 ml, ferric chloride 16 ml, iodine 16
ml. Mallory states that nuclear staining can be
eliminated by doubling the volume of iodine in the
formula.

2.   Differentiating solution. Prepare just before use.

Ferric chloride   2 gm
Distilled water   100 ml

3..   Counterstain. Van Gieson's picro-fuchsin solution.

Solution A   Solution B
Acid fuchsin   1 gm   Saturated aqueous solution
Saturated aqueous   of picric acid (about 1.5%)
picric acid   100 ml

For use, combine 1 ml of solution A with 10 ml of
solution B.

4.   Curtis' counterstain.

Ponceau S (C. I. No. 27195) 1% aqueous   10 ml
Picric acid   1% aqueous   86 ml
Acetic acid   1% aqueous   4 ml

PROCEDURE

1.   Deparaffinize and hydrate sections.
2.   It is not necessary to remove mercury crystals be-
      fore staining, mercurial precipitates are removed
      by the staining solution.
3.   Place the sections in Verhoeff's working solution
      for 15 minutes or more until perfectly black.
4.   Differentiate in 2% solution of ferric chloride (in
      a Coplin jar by gently rocking the slide back and
      forth). To observe the stages of differentiation
      the sections may be examined in water under low mag-
      nification. At first look for a large vessel with
      good elastic fibers as a control, then check the
      finer elastic fibers so that they will not be over-
      differentiated.* If differentiation has been carried

*This is the critical part of the method.

too far the sections may be restained provided that they have not been treated with alcohol.

5. Wash in tap water for 5 minutes.
6. Place in 95% alcohol for 30 minutes to remove the iodine stain from the background. If pressed for time, 5% sodium thiosulfate may be substituted for 5 minutes.
7. Rinse in water.
8. Counterstain in Van Gieson's picro-fuchsin solution or Curtis' picro-Ponceau solution for 5 minutes. Agitate slides for 15 seconds.
9. Dehydrate Van Gieson in absolute alcohol, two changes, 1 to 2 minutes each. Curtis in 95% alcohol, then absolute alcohol.
10. Clear in xylene, two changes.
11. Mount in Permount.

Results.   Elastic and degenerated fitsue: black. Nuclei: black. Collagen: red. Muscle cells, fibrin, and glial tissue: yellow.

Note.   Curtis' counterstain is said to be more resistant to fading than Van Gieson' solution.

Ref.   Verhoeff, F.H., J.A.M., 50: (1908), 876-877
            Van Gieson, I., N.Y. State J. Med., 50: (1889), 57-60.
            Curtis, F., C.R. Soc. Biol. Paris., 58: (1905), 1038-1040

ORCEIN STAIN FOR ELASTICA

Fixation.   10% formalin, alcohol or Helly's fluid.

SOLUTIONS

1.   Orcein solution.*

     Orcein   1 gm
     70% alcohol   100 ml
     Concentrated hydrochloric acid   0.6 ml

     Dissolve the orcein in the alcohol then add the hydrochloric acid.

*Orcein, Roboz Surgical Instrument Co., Washington, D. C.

2.   Acid alcohol.

      1% hydrochloric acid in 70% alcohol

3.   Van Gieson's picro-fuchsin.

      Solution A   Solution B
      Acid fuchsin   1 gm   Saturated aqueous solution
      Saturated aqueous   of picric acid (about 1.5%)
      picric acid   100 ml

      To use, combine 1 ml of solution A with 10 ml of
      solution B.

PROCEDURE

   1. Deparaffinize and hydrate formalin and alcohol-fixed
       tissue to 70% alcohol, Helly's to water.
   2. Remove mercury crystals if necessary. Rinse in 70%
       alcohol.
   3. Stain in acid orcein solution for 30 to 60 minutes
       in covered Coplin jar. Does not overstain.
   4. Rinse in distilled water for 2 to 3 minutes.
   5. Wipe off excess water and dip into 95% alcohol to re-
       move excess dye.
   6. Decolorize in absolute alcohol for 5 to 30 minutes.
       The sections should be a pale brown with purple to
       black elastic fibers when seen under the low power
       of the microscope.
   7. Decolorize background in acid alcohol until nearly
       colorless for 2 to 10 minutes. This should be
       carefully controlled under microscope.
   8. Wash in tap water for 5 to 10 minutes.
   9. Counterstain in Van Gieson's picro-fuchsin for 1 to
       2 minutes each.
  10. Rinse in absolute alcohol, two changes, 1 to 2
       minutes each.
  11. Clear in xylene, two changes.
  12. Mount in Permount.

Results. Elastica: deep brown to black. Collagen: red.

Note.   Instead of picro-fuchsin, sections may be
           counterstained with hematoxylin and eosin.

Ref.   McManus, J. F. A. and Mowry, R. W., Staining
           methods Histologic and Histochemical, Harper &
           Row, New York, 1963, pp. 239-240.

PINKUS ACID ORCEIN-GIEMSA METHOD

Fixation. 10% formalin, Helly's or Zenker's fluids.

SOLUTIONS

1. Orcein solution*

    Orcein   1 gm
    70% alcohol   100 ml
    Concentrated hydrochloric acid   0.6 ml

    Dissolve the orcein in the alcohol, then add the
    hydrochloric acid.

2. Acid alcohol.

    Hydrochloric acid   1 ml
    70% alcohol   99 ml

3. Giemsa solution.

    Giemsa stock solution†   5 drops
    Distilled water   100 ml

4. Alcoholic eosin.

    Eosin Y   5 gm
    95% alcohol   100 ml

PROCEDURE

1. Deparaffinize and hydrate sections.
2. Remove mercury crystals if necessary. Rinse in 70%
    alcohol.
3. Stain in acid orcein solution for 30 to 60 minutes
    in covered Coplin jar. Does not overstain.
4. Rinse in distilled water for 2 to 3 minutes.
5. Wipe off excess water and dip into 95% alcohol to re-
    move excess dye.
6. Decolorize in absolute alcohol for 5 to 30 minutes.
    The section should be a pale brown with purple to
    black elastic fibers when seen under the low power
    of the microscope.

*Orcen, Roboz Surgical Instrument Co., Washington, D. C.
†Giemsa stock solution, Gradwold Laboratories, St. Louis,
  Mo. Lillie formula: J. Lab. Clin. Med., 28 (1943), 15.

7. Decolorize background in acid alcohol until nearly
    colorless for 2 to 10 minutes. This should be care-
    fully controlled under microscope.
8. Wash in tap water for 5 to 10 minutes.
9. Stain in dilute Giemsa solution for 2 hours to over-
    night.
10. Blot off excess stain with fine filter paper.
11. Differentiate in 95% alcohol to which a few drops of
    alcoholic eosin have been added until most of the
    blue stain is removed from the connective tissue.
    (Check under microscope.)
12. Dehydrate in absolute alcohol, two changes, 1 to 2
    minutes each.
13. Clear in xylene, two changes.
14. Mount in Permount.

Results.   Nuclei: deep blue. Elastica: deep brown to
            black. Collagen: pink to pale blue. Melanin:
            green to brown. Eosinophilic granules: bright
            red. Mast cell granules: blue to purple.

Note.   McManus and Mowry point out that this method is
            valuable to demonstrate allergic lesions of the
            skin.

Ref.   Pinkus, H., Arch. Dermat. Syph., 49 (1944),
            355-356.

WEIGERT'S STAIN TO DEMONSTRATE ELASTIC FIBERS

Fixation.   10% formalin or Bouin's fluid. Helly's or
            Zenker's may be used, but the results are not
            as brilliant.

SOLUTIONS

1. Weigert's resorcin fuchsin.*

        Basic fuchsin   2 gm
        Resorcin (Resorcinol)†   4 gm
        Distilled water   200 ml
        29% aqueous ferric chloride   25 ml
        95% alcohol   200 ml
        Hydrochloric acid   4 ml

*Resorcin-fuchsin (prepared) Roboz Surgical Instrument
 Co., Washington, D. C.
†Resorcinol, Fisher Scientific Co.

Bring the fuchsin, resorcin, and distilled water to a brisk boil in a porcelain dish. Add the 29% ferric chloride. Stir and boil for 2 to 5 minutes. A precipitate forms. Cool and filter. Discard the filtrate. Leave the precipitate on the filter paper until all the water has drained away. Place in the 60°C oven overnight. Return the filter paper with the precipitate to the porcelain dish which should be dry but may contain whatever part of the precipitate still adheres to it. Add 200 ml of 95% alcohol and heat very carefully, stirring constantly, remove the filter paper from the dish as the precipitate is dissolved off. Cool, filter, and add 95% alcohol to make up the solution to 200 ml. Add 4 ml of hydrochloric acid. The solution keeps well for several months and may be used over and over.

2.   1% hydrochloric acid in 95% alcohol.

3.   Harris' hematoxylin.

Hematoxylin crystals	5 gm
Absolute ethyl alcohol	50 ml
Aluminum and potassium sulfate	
(potassium alum)	100 gm
Mercuric oxide (red)	2.5 gm
Distilled water	1000 ml

Dissolve the hematoxylin in the alcohol, the alum in the water with the aid of gentle heat. Mix the two solutions together and bring to a boil. Withdraw the flame, slowly and carefully add the mercuric oxide. Heat gently and allow to boil for 5 minutes. Place the flask in cold water and cool quickly. Filter and add 40 ml of glacial acetic acid to improve the nuclear staining. Filter the solution each time before use; solution is effective for 1 to 2 months.

4.   Van Gieson's picro-fuchsin counterstain.

Solution A		Solution B
Acid fuchsin	1 gm	Saturated aqueous solution
Saturated aqueous		of picric acid (about 1.5%)
picric acid	100 ml	

For use, combine 1 ml of solution A with 10 ml of solution B.

PROCEDURE

1. Deparaffinize and hydrate sections.
2. Remove mercury crystals if necessary.
3. Stain in resorcin-fuchsin solution for 20 minutes to 1 hour. Control under microscope and stain until the elastic fibers are black.
4. Wash in several changes of 95% alcohol to remove excess stain.
5. If excess stain is present, differentiate in acid alcohol solution (solution 2).
6. Wash in tap water.
7. If a counterstain is desired, stain in Harris' hematoxylin as usual, followed by Van Gieson's picrofuchsin.
8. Differentiate and dehydrate in absolute alcohol, two changes, 1 to 2 minutes each.
9. Clear in xylene, two changes.
10. Mount in Permount.

Results.   Elastic fibers are stained dark blue to black. If Van Gieson's counterstain and nuclear stain are used, nuclei appear black, collagen red, muscle, fibrin and neuroglia fibers yellow.

Ref.   Mallory, F. B., Pathological Technique, Hafner Publishing Co., New York, 1968.

FULMER'S AND LILLIE'S ORCINOL-NEW FUCHSIN   ELASTIC FIBER STAIN

Fixation. 10% formalin, Helly's fluid.

SOLUTIONS

1.   New fuchsin   2 gm
      Orcinol*   4 gm
      Distilled water   200 ml

      Boil for 5 minutes and add 25 ml of Liquor Ferri Chloridi U. S. P. 1X and boil for 5 minutes more. [15.5 gm of ferric chloride (lump) $FeCL_3.6 H_2O$ and water to make up 25 ml may be substituted if U. S. P. is not available.] Cool, collect precipitate on filter paper, and dissolve it in 100 ml of 95% alcohol. This is the working solution.

*Orcinol, Fisher Scientific Co.

2.   Van Gieson's picro-fuchsin solution.

Solution A   Solution B
Acid fuchsin   1 gm Saturated aqueous solution
Saturated aqueous   of picric acid (about 1.5%)
picric acid   100 ml

For use, combine 1 ml of solution A with 10 ml of
solution B.

PROCEDURE

1.   Deparaffinize sections to absolute alcohol.
2.   Stain in the orcinol-new fuchsin solution for 15
     minutes at 37°C.
3.   Differentiate in three changes of 70% alcohol, 5 min-
     utes each.
4.   Counterstain if desired in Van Gieson's picro-fuch-
     sin, 2 to 5 minutes. Agitate slides in solution for
     15 seconds.
5.   Dehydrate in absolute alcohol, two changes, 1 to 2
     minutes each.
6.   Clear in xylene, two changes.
7.   Mount in Permount.

Results.   Elastic fibers: deep violet. Other tissue ele-
           ments: unstained or depend on counterstain.

Ref.   Fulmer, H. M., and Lillie, R.D., Stain Tech.,
           31 (1956), 27-29. Copyright the Williams and
           Wilkins Co.

GOMORI'S ALDEHYDE-FUCHSIN ELASTIC FIBER STAIN

Fixation.   10% formalin, Helly's or Bouin's fluids. 10%
            formalin or Bouin's fluid give colorless back-
            grounds.

SOLUTIONS

1.   Gomori's aldehyde fuchsin.

Basic fuchsin   1 gm
70% alcohol   200 ml
Concentrated hydrochloric acid   2 ml
Paraldehyde   2 ml

Add the hydrochloric acid and the paraldehyde to the
basic fuchsin solution. Let stand at room tempera-

ture for 2 to 3 days until a deep purple color develops. Store in refrigerator. Filter and allow to
warm to room temperature before using. Does not
keep well.

2.   Van Gieson's picro-fuchsin counterstain.

Solution A   Solution B
Acid fuchsin   1 gm   Saturated aqueous solution
Saturated aqueous   of picric acid (about 1.5%)
picric acid   100 ml

For use, combine 1 ml of solution A with 10 ml of
solution B.

PROCEDURE

1.   Deparaffinize and hydrate sections.
2.   Remove mercury crystals if necessary.
3.   Wash well in water.
4.   Rinse in several changes of 70% alcohol.
5.   Stain in aldehyde-fuchsin for 5 to 10 minutes in
      covered Coplin jar.
6.   Rinse in three changes of 70% alcohol to remove ex-
      cess stain.
7.   Rinse in distilled water; check for blue elastic
      fibers.
8.   Counterstain in Van Gieson for 1 minute. Agitate
      slides in solution.
9.   Differentiate and dehydrate in two changes of abso-
      lute alcohol 1 to 2 minutes each.
10.   Clear in xylene, two changes.
11.   Mount in Permount.

Results.   Elastic fibers and mucin: blue. Collagen: red.
           Mast cells: blue.

Note.   If overcounterstained, water will remove Van
           Gieson's picro-fuchsin. To demonstrate pan-
           creatic islet cells, stain for 15 to 30 minutes;
           pituitary beta cell granules, 30 minutes to 2
           hours.

Ref.   Gomori, G., Amer. J. Clin. Path., 20 (1950),
           665-666.

PUTT AND HUKILL COMBINED MUCIN AND ELASTIC TISSUE METHOD

<u>Fixation</u>. 10% formalin, Helly or Zenker's fluids.

SOLUTIONS

1. Alcian green.

Alcian green 2 GX or 3 BX	1 gm
Distilled water	100 ml
Glacial acetic acid	2 ml

    Add a crystal of thymol as a preservative. Filter before use.

2. Verhoeff's elastic tissue solutions.

    A. | Hematoxylin | 5 gm |
        |---|---|
        | Absolute alcohol | 100 ml |

    Dissolve the hematoxylin in the alcohol with the aid of gentle heat (water bath). Cool, filter, and store in a tightly stoppered bottle.

    B. Verhoeff's iodine solution.

Iodine crystals	2 gm
Potassium iodide	4 gm
Distilled water	100 ml

    Dissolve the potassium iodide in a small portion of distilled water, add the iodine, shake well, and then add the balance of the distilled water.

    C. Ferric chloride solution

Ferric chloride	10 gm
Distilled water	100 ml

    D. Working solution. Combine in order given.
Solution A	60 ml
Solution B	24 ml
Solution C	24 ml

    Filter before use. The combined solution is stable for about 24 hours.

3.   Differentiating solution.   Prepare just before use.

      Ferric chloride   2 gm
      Distilled water   100 ml

4.   Van Gieson's picro-fuchsin counterstain.

      Solution A   Solution B
      Acid fuchsin   1 gm   Saturated aqueous picric
      Saturated aqueous   acid (about 1 to 1.5%)
      picric acid   100 ml

      For use, combine 1 ml of solution A with 10 ml of
      solution B.

PROCEDURE

1.   Deparaffinize and hydrate sections.
2.   Remove mercury crystals if necessary.
3.   Stain in freshly filtered alcian green for 10 minutes.
4.   Rinse in distilled water.
5.   Stain in freshly filtered Verhoeff's elastic stain
     for 15 to 30 minutes.
6.   Differentiate in 2% ferric chloride (in a Coplin
     jar by gently rocking the slide back and forth).
     To observe the stages of differentiation the sec-
     tions may be examined in water under low magnifica-
     tion. At first look for a vessel with good elastic
     fibers as a control, then check the finer elastic
     fibers so that they will not be overdifferentiated.
     If differentiation has been carried too far, the
     sections may be restained provided they have not
     been treated with alcohol.
7.   Wash in tap water for 5 minutes.
8.   Place in 95% alcohol for 30 minutes to remove the
     iodine stain from the background.
9.   Rinse in water.
10. Counterstain in Van Gieson's picro-fuchsin for 5
     minutes. Agitate slides for 15 seconds.
11. Dehydrate in absolute alcohol, two changes, 1 to 2
     minutes each.
12. Clear in xylene, two changes.
13. Mount in Permount.

Results. Mucin and connective tissue mucopolysaccharides:
          green. Elastic fibers: black. Nuclei: blue to
          black. Collagen: red. Other tissue elements:
          yellow.

Ref.   Putt, F.A., and Hukill, P.B., A.M.A. Arch.
              Path., 74 (1962), 169-170 Copyright American
              Medical Association.

MAYER'S MUCICARMINE STAIN

Fixation. Helly's fluid (Zenker-formol) preferred; other
           fixatives may be used.

SOLUTIONS

1.   Harris' hematoxylin.

      Hematoxylin crystals   5 gm
      Absolute ethyl alcohol   50 ml
      Aluminum and potassium sulfate
      (potassium alum)   100 gm
      Mercuric oxide (red)   2.5 gm
      Distilled water   1000 ml

      Dissolve the hematoxylin in the alcohol, the alum in
      water with the aid of heat. Mix the two solutions
      together and bring to a boil. Withdraw the flame,
      slowly and carefully add the mercuric oxide, heat
      gently, and allow to continue to boil for 5 minutes.
      Place the flask in cold water and cool quickly. Fil-
      ter and add 40 ml of glacial acetic acid to improve
      nuclear staining. Filter the solution each time be-
      fore use. Solution effective for 1 to 2 months.

2.   Mayer's mucicarmine solution (stock solution).

      Carmine (alum lake) (C. I. No. 75470)   1 gm
      Aluminum chloride (anhydrous)   0.5 gm
      Distilled water   2 ml

      Combine and heat in a porcelain dish over a small
      flame for 2 minutes, stirring constantly with a
      glass rod until the reddish mixture becomes a dark
      color. Remove from flame and gradually add, stir-
      ring constantly, 100 ml of 50% alcohol. Let stand
      for 24 hours in a covered dish, then filter. Stock
      solution keeps well.

PROCEDURE

1.   Deparaffinize and hydrate sections. (Use control
      slide.)
2.   Remove mercury crystals if necessary.

3.   Stain nuclei in Harris' hematoxylin if nuclear de-
      tail is desired.
4.   Stain in Mayer's dilute mucicarmine for 10 to 30
      minutes.
      Working solution: 1 part of stock solution with 10
      parts of 60% alcohol. (Discard diluted solution.)
5.   Wash quickly in distilled water.
6.   Dehydrate in 95% alcohol, then absolute alcohol, two
      changes, 1 to 2 minutes each.
7.   Clear in xylene, two changes.
8.   Mount in Permount.

Results. Mucin: red. Nuclei: blue, if stained.

Ref.   Mallory, F. B., Pathological Technique, Hafner
          Publishing Co., New York, 1968.

MASSON'S MODIFICATION OF MAYER'S MUCICARMINE STAIN

Fixation. Absolute alcohol. 10% formalin may be used
          provided that is not alkaline. The addi-
          tion of 5% acetic acid is advised. After
          formalin fixation for 12 to 24 hours the tissue
          should be preserved in 80% alchhol/

SOLUTIONS

1.   Mayer's hemalum.

      Hematoxylin crystals   1 gm
      Sodium iodate   0.2 gm
      Aluminum and ammonium sulfate
      (ammonia alum)   50 gm
      Distilled water   1000 ml
      Chloral hydrate   50 gm
      Citric acid   1 gm

      Dissolve hematoxylin, sodium iodate, and the ammo-
      nia alum overnight in 1000 ml of distilled water;
      add the chloral hydrate and citric acid. Boil for
      5 minutes; when cool, it is ready for use. The solu-
      tion keeps well.

2.   Metanil yellow.

      Metanil yellow   0.05 gm
      Acetic acid water (acetic acid 1 ml;
      distilled water 500 ml)   100 ml

3.   Mayer's mucicarmine (stock solution).

Carmine alum lake (C. I. No. 75470)   1 gm
Aluminum chloride   0.5 gm
Distilled water   2 gm

Combine and heat in a porcelain dish over a small
flame for 2 minutes, stirring constantly with a
glass rod until the mixture takes on a dark color.
Remove from the flame and gradually add with constant stirring 100 ml of 50% alcohol. Cover well,
let stand for 24 hours, and filter. Stock solution
keeps well.

4.   Mayer's mucicarmine working solution.

Stock solution   2 ml
Tap water   20 ml

Make up just sufficient solution to stain slides
being processed. Discard diluted solution.

PROCEDURE

1.   Deparaffinize and hydrate sections. (Use a control
      slide.)
2.   Stain in Mayer's hemalum for 5 minutes. Do not
      differentiate; the mucicarmine which is slightly
      acid will do it.
3.   Wash in water.
4.   Stain in metanil yellow for 30 seconds to 1 minute.
5.   Rinse in distilled water. (Background should be
      yellow.)
6.   Stain in mucicarmine working solution for 1 to 3
      hours at room temperature.
7.   Rinse in distilled water.
8.   Dehydrate in 95% alcohol, then absolute alcohol, two
      changes, 1 to 2 minutes each.
9.   Clear in xylene, two changes.
10.   Mount in Permount.

Results.   The mucus of the Goblet cells of the intestine,
           fundamental substance of cartilage: dark violet
           red. Cytoplasm and collagen fibers: yellow.
           Nuclei: blue-black. In man, the mucus of the
           superficial cells of the stomach remain yellow.

Ref.   Masson, P., personal communication.

PUTT AND HUKILL ALCIAN GREEN METHOD FOR MUCINS

Fixation.   10% formalin, Helly's or Zenker's fluids.

SOLUTIONS

1.   Alcian green.*

Alcian green 2 GX or 3 BX	0.1 gm
Distilled water	100 ml
Glacial acetic acid	2 ml

Add a crystal of thymol as a preservative. Filter
before use.

2.   Nuclear fast red (Kernechtrot).†

Nuclear fast red	1 gm
Aluminum sulfate	5 gm
Distilled water	100 ml

Dissolve the nuclear fast red in the aluminum sulfate solution. Bring to a boil, cool, and filter.

3.   Metanil yellow counterstain.

Metanil yellow	0.25 gm
Distilled water	100 ml
Glacial acetic acid	2 drops

PROCEDURE

1.   Deparaffinize and hydrate sections. (Use control
     slide.)
2.   Remove mercury crystals if necessary.
3.   Stain in freshly filtered alcian green for 10 min-
     utes.
4.   Rinse in distilled water.
5.   Stain nuclei in nuclear fast red for 5 to 10 min-
     utes. Overstaining rarely occurs, but Helly, Zen-
     ker, or corrosive sublimate fixatives stain more
     rapidly than formalin-fixed material.
6.   Rinse in distilled water.
7.   Counterstain in metanil yellow for 1/2 minute.

---

*Alcian green, ESBE Laboratory Supplies, Toronto, Ontario,
 Canada.
†Nuclear fast red (Kernechtrot), Roboz Surgical Instru-
 ment Co., Washington, D. C.

8.   Rinse well in distilled water.
9.   Dehydrate in 95% alcohol, then in absolute alcohol,
     two changes, 1 to 2 minutes each.
10. Clear in xylene, two changes.
11. Mount in Permount.

Results.   Muchin: green. Nuclei: red. Backgroung: yellow.

Ref.   Putt, F.A. and Hukill, P.B., A.M.A. Arch. Path.,
           74 (1962), 169-170. Copyright American Medical
           Association

ATTWOOD'S ALCIAN GREEN-PHLOXINE METHOD TO
DEMONSTRATE EPITHELIAL SQUAMES

Fixation.   10% formol saline, saturated aqueous mercuric
            chloride, Helly's and Bouin's fluids.

SOLUTIONS

1.   Alcian green solution.*

     Alcian green 2 GX   1 gm
     Glacial acetic acid   2 ml
     Distilled water   98 ml

     Add a crystal of thymol as a preservative.

2.   Potassium permanganate.

     Potassium permanganate   0.5 gm
     Distilled water   100 ml

3.   Oxalic acid.

     Oxalic acid   5 gm
     Distilled water   100 ml

4.   Mayer's hemalum.

     Hematoxylin crystals   1 gm
     Sodium iodate   0.2 gm
     Aluminum and ammonium sulfate
     (ammonia alum)   50 gm
     Distilled water   1000 ml
     Chloral hydrate   50 gm
     Citric acid   1 gm

*Alcian green 2 GX, ESBE Laboratory Supplies, Toronto,
Ontario, Canada.

Dissolve hematoxylin, sodium iodate, and the ammonia alum overnight in 1000 ml of distilled water. Add the chloral hydrate and citric acid. Boil for 5 minutes; when cool, it is ready for use. The solution keeps well.

5.   Scott's tap water substitute.

Sodium bicarbonate	2 gm
Magnesium sulfate	20 gm
Distilled water	1000 ml

6.   Phloxine solution.

Phloxine	0.5 gm
Calcium chloride	0.5 gm
Distilled water	100 ml

Filter before use each time.

7.   Cellosolve.*

8.   Tartrazine solution.†

Tartrazine	2 gm
Cellosolve	100 ml

Heat in a water bath to form a saturated solution, cool, and filter.

PROCEDURE

1.   Deparaffinize and hydrate sections.
2.   Remove mercury crystals if necessary.
3.   Stain in alcian green solution for 5 minutes.
4.   Rinse in tap water.
5.   Place in potassium permanganate for 2 minutes.
6.   Rinse in tap water.
7.   Place in oxalic acid for 5 minutes.
8.   Wash in tap water.
9.   Stain in Mayer's hemalum for 5 minutes.
10. Rinse in tap water.
11. Blue in Scott's tap water substitute for 5 minutes.
12. Rinse in tap water.
13. Stain in phloxine solution for 15 to 30 minutes.

*Cellosolve: ethylene glycol monoethyl ether.

†Tartrazine: ESBE Laboratory Supplies, Toronto, Ontario, Canada.

14.   Rinse in tap water.
15.   Rinse in Cellosolve.
16.   Differentiate sections individually with constant
      agitation, in tartrazine-cellosolve solution, check-
      ing with the low power of the microscope until the
      phloxine is removed from the red cells. Any excess
      staining with the tartrazine can be removed by
      rinsing in water until the desired intensity is ob-
      tained.
17.   Dehydrate in Cellosolve, two changes.
18.   Clear in xylene, two changes.
19.   Mount in Permount.

Results.   Nuclei: blue-black. Ground substance of carti-
           lage, mucin, and the granules of certain mast
           cells: green. Epithelial squames and fibrin:
           red. Erythrocytes, plasma, and collagen: yellow.

Note.   Steps 5 to 7 are not strictly necessary, but
           they assist in the subsequent differentiation
           of the phloxine and tend to remove any back-
           ground staining by the alcian green.

Ref.   Attwood, H. D., J. Path. Bact., 76 (1958), 211-
           215.

PUTT'S ALCIAN GREEN-CALCIUM CHLORIDE METHOD TO
DEMONSTRATE MUCINS

Fixation.   10% formalin, Helly's fluid or any routine
            fixative.

SOLUTIONS

1.   Celestin blue. Dissolve 5 gm of ferric ammonium
      sulfate (iron alum) overnight at room temperature
      in 100 ml of distilled water. Bring to a boil, add
      0.5 gm of celestin blue, and boil carefully for 3
      minutes. Filter, cool, and add 14 ml of glycerin.
      The solution keeps well at room temperature. Filter
      before use.

2.   Mayer's hemalum.

      Hematoxylin crystals   1 gm
      Sodium iodate   0.2 gm
      Aluminum and ammonium sulfate
      (ammonia alum)   50 gm

Distilled water	1000 ml
Chloral hydrate	50 gm
Citric acid	1 gm

Dissolve hematoxylin, sodium iodate, and the ammonia alum overnight in 1000 ml of distilled water. Add the chloral hydrate and citric acid. Boil for 5 minutes; when cool, it is ready for use. The solution keeps well.

3. Alcian green 2 GX solution.*

Alcian green 2 GX	1 gm
Calcium chloride ($CaCl_2 \cdot 2H_2O$)	0.5 gm
Distilled water	100 ml

Dissolve the calcium chloride in the water, then add the dye. Add a crystal of thymol as a preservative. Filter before use. Solution keeps well.

4. Martius yellow counterstain.

Dissolve 0.5 gm of martius yellow in 20 ml of distilled water and 1 gm of phosphomolybdic acid in 80 ml of absolute alcohol. Combine and filter.

Solution keeps well at room temperature.

PROCEDURE

1. Deparaffinize and hydrate sections. (Use control slide.)
2. Remove mercury crystals if necessary.
3. Stain in celestin blue for 5 minutes.
4. Wash in tap water for 2 to 3 minutes.
5. Stain in Mayer's hemalum for 5 minutes.
6. Wash well in tap water.
7. Differentiate nuclei in acid alcohol for a few seconds (1 ml of hydrochloric acid in 99 ml of 70% alcohol).
8. Wash in running tap water for 5 minutes.
9. Stain in alcian green 2 GX for 5 minutes.
10. Rinse in distilled water.
11. Counterstain in Martius yellow for 15 to 30 seconds.
12. Rinse in tap water.

*Alcian Green 2 GX, ESBE Laboratory Supplies, Toronto, Ontario, Canada.

13. Dehydrate in 95% alcohol then absolute alcohol, two
    changes, 1 to 2 minutes each.
14. Clear in xylene.
15. Mount in Permount.

Results.   Nuclei: blue-black. Connective tissue muco-
            polysaccharides, mucin, and ground substance
            of cartilage: green. Erythrocytes, muscle,
            and fibrous tissue: yellow. Mast cell granules
            and cryptococcus are also demonstrated.

Ref.   Putt, F. A., Yale J. Biol. Med., 43 (1971),
            279-282.

PIOCH'S ASTRA BLUE METHOD TO DEMONSTRATE
ACID MUCOPOLYSACCHARIDES

Fixation.   10% formalin.

SOLUTIONS

1.   Astra blue solution.*

     Astra blue   1 gm
     Distilled water   100 ml
     Tartaric acid   2-3 gm

2.   Nuclear fast red counterstain.

     Nuclear fast red (Kernechtrot)   0.1 gm
     Aluminum sulfate   5 gm
     Distilled water   100 ml

     Dissolve the nuclear fast red in the aluminum sul-
     fate solution, bring to a boil, cool, and filter.
     Solution keeps well at room temperature.

PROCEDURE

1.   Deparaffinize and hydrate sections. (Use control
     slide.)
2.   Stain in astra blue for 5 to 10 minutes.
3.   Rinse in distilled water.
4.   Counterstain in nuclear fast red for 5 to 10 minutes.
5.   Rinse in distilled water.

*Astra blue, Roboz Surgical Instrument Co., Washington, D.C.

6.   Dehydrate in 95% alcohol then absolute alcohol, two
     changes, 1 to 2 minutes each.
7.   Clear in xylene, two changes.
8.   Mount in Permount.

Results. Acid mucopolysaccharides: blue. Nuclei: red.

Ref.   Pioch, W., Virchow. Archiv., 330 (1957), 337.

MOWRY'S COMBINED ALCIAN BLUE PERIODIC ACID-SCHIFF METHOD

Fixation. 10% formalin, Helly's or Bouin's fluids.

SOLUTIONS

1.   Glacial acetic acid   3 ml
     Distilled water   100 ml

2.   Alcian blue solution.

     Alcian blue 8 GX   1 gm
     Distilled water   97 ml
     Glacial acetic acid   3 ml

     Filter and add a crystal of thymol as a preservative.

3.   Periodic acid   0.5 gm
     Distilled water   100 ml

4.   Normal hydrochloric acid.

     Hydrochloric acid, sp. gr. 1.19   83.5 ml
     Distilled water   916.5 ml

5.   Schiff reagent. Bring 200 ml of distilled water to
     a boil, remove from flame, add 1 gm of basic fuchsin
     and stir until dissolved. Cool to 50°C. Add 1 gm
     of sodium or potassium metabisulfite ($Na_2S_2O_5$,
     $K_2S_2O_5$). Place in the dark in a stoppered bottle
     for 18 to 24 hours. Solution takes on an orange
     color. Add 0.5 gm of activated charcoal and shake
     well, then filter through a coarse filter paper.
     Store under refrigeration in a brown stoppered bottle
     of the same volume. Solution is stable for several
     weeks. Use at room temperature. If a pink color
     develops, discard.

6.   Sulfurous acid rinse.

10% sodium metabisulfite	6 ml
Normal hydrochloric acid	5 ml
Distilled water	100 ml

7.   Harris' hematoxylin.

Hematoxylin crystals	5 gm
Absolute ethyl alcohol	50 ml
Aluminum and potassium sulfate (potassium alum)	100 gm
Mercuric oxide (red)	2.5 gm
Distilled water	1000 ml

      Dissolve the hematoxylin in the alcohol and the alum
      in the water with the aid of gentle heat. Mix the
      two solutions together and bring to a boil. With-
      draw the flame, slowly and carefully add the mercu-
      ric oxide, heat gently, and allow to continue to
      boil for 5 minutes. Place the flask in cold water
      and cool quickly. Filter and add 40 ml of glacial
      acetic acid to improve nuclear staining. Filter
      before use.

8. | | |
      |---|---|
      | Picric acid | 0.5 gm |
      | Distilled water | 100 ml |

PROCEDURE

1. Deparaffinize and hydrate sections.
2. Remove mercury crystals if necessary.
3. Rinse in 3% acetic acid for 3 minutes.
4. Stain in alcian blue solution for 2 hours.
5. Rinse in tap water and place in 3% acetic acid for 3 to 5 minutes.
6. Rinse in running tap water for 3 minutes; rinse in distilled water.
7. Oxidize in periodic acid for 10 minutes.
8. Wash in running tap water for 5 minutes. Rinse in distilled water.
9. Place in Schiff's reagent for 10 minutes.
10. Rinse in sulfurous acid rinse, two changes, 2 minutes each.
11. Wash in running tap water for 5 minutes. Rinse in distilled water.
12. Stain for 5 minutes in Harris' hematoxylin.
13. Wash in running tap water for 3 to 5 minutes.
14. Differentiate in acid alcohol for 2 to 30 seconds (70% alcohol, 99 ml; hydrochloric acid 1 ml).

15. Wash in running tap water for 3 minutes.
16. Optional picric acid background stain: Place in
     picric acid solution for 1 minute, rinse for a few
     seconds in tap water. (When picric acid is used
     omit steps 14 and 15.)
17. Dehydrate in 95% alcohol, then in absolute alcohol,
     two changes, 1 to 2 minutes each.
18. Clear in xylene, two changes.
19. Mount in Permount.

Results.   Complex carbohydrates rich in acidic groups
            (especially carboxyls) mucins of soft connec-
            tive tissue and their tumors, are colored tur-
            quoise blue, while neutral carbohydrates rich
            in vicinal hydroxyl groups, that is, glycogen
            or human Brunner's gland mucin are colored ma-
            genta. Carbohydrates having both acidic groups
            and oxidizable hydroxyl groups, that is, mucins
            of most epithelial cells and their tumors, are
            colored both Alcian blue and PAS, resulting in
            deeper blue to purple shades. Hematoxylin
            stains nuclei reddish brown. When picric acid
            is used, erythrocytes and the cytoplasm of most
            cells are yellow.

Ref.   McManus, J.F.A. and Mowry, R.W. Staining Methods
            Histologic and Histochemical 1963 Harper and Row
            Publishers, Inc Maryland.

MAXWELL'S METHOD TO DEMONSTRATE METAPLASTIC
EPITHELIUM IN THE STOMACH

Fixation. 10% buffered formalin, 10% formalin.

SOLUTIONS

1.   Alcian green 3 BX.

     Alcian green 3 BX.*   1 gm
     Distilled water   100 ml

     Add a crystal of thymol as a preservative.

2.   Periodic acid solution.

     Periodic acid   0.5 gm
     Distilled water   100 ml

*Alcian Green 3 BX, Roboz Surgical Instrument Co.,
Washington, D.C.

3. Normal hydrochloric acid. (Store in refrigerator.)

    Hydrochloric acid, sp. gr. 1.19   83.5 ml
    Distilled water   916.5 ml

4. Sodium metabisulfite (Na2S205)   10 gm
    Distilled water   100 ml

5. Sulfurous acid rinse. Discard after use.

    Normal hydrochloric acid   5 ml
    10% sodium metabisulfite   6 ml
    Distilled water   100 ml

6. Alcian yellow GXS*   1 gm
    Distilled water   100 ml

    Add a crystal of thymol as a preservative.

7. Mayer's hemalum.

    Hematoxylin crystals   1 gm
    Sodium iodate   0.2 gm
    Aluminum and ammonium sulfate
    (ammonia alum)   50 gm
    Distilled water   1000 ml
    Chloral hydrate   50 gm
    Citric acid   1 gm

    Dissolve hematoxylin, sodium iodate, and the ammo-
    nia alum overnight in 1000 ml of distilled water.
    Add the chloral hydrate and citric acid. Boil for
    5 minutes; when cool, it is ready for use. The solu-
    tion keeps well.

PROCEDURE

1. Deparaffinize and hydrate sections. (Run a control
    slide.)
2. Stain in 1% alcian green for 5 minutes.
3. Rinse in water.
4. Place in periodic acid for 5 minutes.
5. Rinse in water.
6. Place in sulfurous acid rinse for 5 minutes, two
    changes. (Discard.)

*Alcian yellow GXS, Roboz Surgical Instrument Co.,
Washington, D.C.

7. Place directly in alcian yellow for 10 to 15 minutes.
8. Rinse in water.
9. Stain nuclei in Mayer's hemalum for 3 to 4 minutes.
10. Wash well in tap water.
11. Dehydrate in 95% alcohol, then absolute alcohol, two
    changes, 1 to 2 minutes each.
12. Clear in xylene, two changes.
13. Mount in Permount.

Results.   Gastric mucin: yellow. Intestinal mucin: green.
           Nuclei: blue.

Ref.   Maxwell, A., Stain Tech., 38 (1963), 286-287.
           Copyright The Williams and Wilkins Co.

MAXWELL'S METHOD TO DEMONSTRATE GASTRIC MUCOUS CELLS

Fixation.   10% formalin, 10% buffered formalin.

SOLUTIONS

1. Periodic acid.

    Periodic acid   0.5 gm
    Distilled water   100 ml

2. Normal hydrochloric acid.   (Store in refrigerator.)

    Hydrochloric acid, sp. gr. 1.19   83.5 ml
    Distilled water   916.5 ml

3. Sodium metabisulfite (Na2S205)   10 gm
    Distilled water   100 ml

4. Sulfurous acid rinse.

    10% sodium metabisulfite   6 ml
    Normal hydrochloric acid   5 ml
    Distilled water   100 ml

5. Alcian green 3 BX solution.

    Alcian green 3 BX   1 gm
    Distilled water   100 ml

    Add a crystal of thymol as a preservative.

6.   Mayer's hemalum.

Hematoxylin crystals	1 gm
Sodium iodate	0.2 gm
Aluminum and ammonium sulfate	
(ammonia alum)	50 gm
Distilled water	1000 ml
Chloral hydrate	50 gm
Citric acid	1 gm

Dissolve hematoxylin, sodium iodate, and the ammonia alum overnight in 1000 ml of distilled water. Add the chloral hydrate and citric acid. Boil for 5 minutes; when cool, it is ready for use. The solution keeps well.

PROCEDURE

1.   Deparaffinize and hydrate sections.   (Run a control slide.)
2.   Place in periodic acid for 5 minutes.
3.   Wash briefly in water.
4.   Place in sulfurous acid rinse solution for 5 minutes, two changes.   (Discard.)
5.   Place directly in alcian green solution for 10 to 15 minutes.
6.   Rinse 2 to 3 seconds in water.
7.   Stain nuclei in Mayer's hemalum 3 to 4 minutes.
8.   Wash well in tap water.
9.   Dehydrate in 95% alcohol, then in absolute alcohol, two changes, 1 to 2 minutes each.
10. Clear in xylene, two changes.
11. Mount in Permount.

Results.   Gastric mucin: green.   Nuclei: blue.

Ref.   Maxwell, A., Stain Tech., 38 (1963), 286-287. Copyright The Williams and Wilkins Co.

PERIODIC ACID-SCHIFF REACTION

Fixation.   10% formalin, Helly's fluid.

SOLUTIONS

1.   Periodic acid.*

*Periodic acid, The G. Frederick Smith Chemical Co., Columbus, Ohio.

Periodic acid crystals   0.5 gm
Distilled water   100 ml

2. Hydrochloric acid, sp. gr. 1.19   83.5 ml
    Distilled water   916.5 ml

3. Schiff reagent. Bring 200 ml of distilled water to
    a boil, remove from flame, and add 1 gm of basic
    fuchsin and stir until dissolved. Cool to 50°C.
    Filter and add 20 ml of normal hydrochloric acid.
    Cool further to 25°C. Add 1 gm of sodium or potas-
    sium metabisulfite (Na2S205 K2S205). Place in the
    dark in a stoppered bottle for 18 to 24 hours; solu-
    tion takes on an orange color. Add 0.5 gm of acti-
    vated charcoal and shake well, then filter through
    a coarse filter paper. Store under refrigeration
    in a brown stoppered bottle of the same volume.
    Solution is stable for several weeks. Use at room
    temperature.

4. Sodium bisulfite   10 gm
    Distilled water   100 ml

5. Sulfurous acid rinse. (Discard after use.)

    10% sodium metabisulfite (Na2S205)   6 ml
    Normal hydrochloric acid   5 ml
    Distilled water   100 ml

6. Harris' hematoxylin.

    Hematoxylin crystals   5 gm
    Absolute ethyl alcohol   50 ml
    Aluminum and potassium sulfate
    (potassium alum)   100 gm
    Mercuric oxide (red)   2.5 gm
    Distilled water   1000 ml

    Dissolve the hematoxylin in the alcohol and the alum
    in the water with the aid of heat. Mix the two
    solutions together and bring to a boil. Withdraw
    the flame, slowly and carefully add the mercuric
    oxide. Heat gently and allow to continue to boil
    for 5 minutes. Place the flask in cold water and
    cool quickly. Filter and add 40 ml of glacial ace-
    tic acid to improve nuclear staining. Filter the
    solution each time before use. Solution effective
    for 1 to 2 months.

PROCEDURE

1. Deparaffinize and hydrate sections. (Run a control slide.)
2. Remove mercury crystals if necessary.
3. Rinse in distilled water. (See digestion note.)
4. Place in periodic acid solution for 5 minutes.
5. Rinse in distilled water.
6. Place in Schiff's reagent for 15 minutes.
7. Rinse in three changes of sulfurous acid rinse for 2 minutes each. If running a number of slides, change the solutions as they become pink.
8. Wash in running tap water for 10 minutes.
9. Counterstain lightly in Harris' hematoxylin, 30 seconds. (If overstained, the magenta color reaction of the Schiff reagent will appear purple.) (Lillie advises the elimination of all counterstains for critical histochemistry.)
10. Wash in tap water.
11. Dehydrate in 95% alcohol, then in absolute alcohol, two changes, 1 to 2 minutes each.
12. Clear in xylene, two changes.
13. Mount in Permount.

Results. Carbohydrates and PAS positive material such as glycogen, mucin, hyaline deposits in glomeruli, and basement membranes stain magenta to purple. Amyloid may show a positive reaction. Nuclei stain blue.

Note. If digestion is required (step 3), place sections in a 1% aqueous (distilled water) solution of diastase for 1 to 2 hours at room temperature. Wash in running tap water, then in distilled water before going into periodic acid. Tissues containing glycogen that have been fixed in solutions with picric acid are slightly more resistant to digestion.

If the Schiff reagent takes on a pink or red color, it is no longer effective. Schiff reagent should turn reddish purple rapidly if added to a small amount of 40% formaldehyde in a dish. If the reaction is slow and the color is blue-purple, replace the solution. New solutions should always be tested with a control slide. Some samples of basic fuchsin are not suitable to prepare Schiff solution; if a good sample is found it should be reserved for this purpose. The solution is best prepared fresh each month.

Overstained sections may be decolorized in 5% aqueous solution of chlorox. Rinse in water.

Stain may be removed by treating sections in 0.5% potassium permanganate for 5 minutes. Wash in water for 5 minutes and place in 5% aqueous oxalic acid for 5 minutes. Wash well in water.

JONES' MODIFICATION OF THE METHENAMINE SILVER STAIN TO DEMONSTRATE THE FINER STRUCTURES OF GLOMERULAR CONNECTIVE TISSUE

Fixation.   10% formalin, Carnoy's, Bouin's fluids. Mer-
            cury-containing fixatives result in a granular
            stain.

SOLUTIONS

1.   Periodic acid   0.5 gm
     Distilled water   100 ml

2.   Silver nitrate   5 gm
     Distilled water   100 ml

3.   Methenamine   3 gm
     Distilled water   100 ml

4.   Borax (sodium borate)   5 gm
     Distilled water   100 ml

5.   Stock methenamine silver solution.

     Methenamine 3%   100 ml
     Silver nitrate 5%   5 ml

A white precipitate appears but immediately dissolves on shaking. The clear solution lasts for months if kept refrigerated.

6.   Methenamine working solution.

     Borax 5%   2 ml
     Distilled water   25 ml
     Stock methenamine silver solution   25 ml

7. Toning solution.

    1/500 yellow gold chloride

8. Sodium thiosulfate   2 gm
    Distilled water   100 ml

9. Masson's trichrome stain.

PROCEDURE

1. Cut paraffin sections at 2 to 3 microns.
2. Deparaffinize and hydrate to distilled water.
3. Place sections in periodic acid at room temperature
    for 15 minutes.
4. Rinse well in distilled water.
5. Place in methenamine silver solution at 45 to 50°C
    for 1 1/2 to 3 hours. (Jones, personal communica-
    tion, now stains for 45 minutes in a 60°C water
    bath.) Sections may be rinsed in distilled water
    and examined under the microscope. If further stain-
    ing is necessary, rinse in distilled water and re-
    place in silver solution. If staining is too in-
    tense, rinse briefly in a very dilute solution of
    potassium ferricyanide, then rinse in distilled
    water. Do not use metallic forceps in silver solu-
    tion.
6. Wash in distilled water.
7. Tone in yellow gold chloride for 2 to 3 minutes.
    (Discard.)
8. Wash in distilled water.
9. Fix in sodium thiosulfate for 2 minutes.
10. Wash well in tap water.
11. We now do a complete Masson stain. The nuclear
    stain in celestin blue and Mayer's hemalum should be
    slightly increased. Hematoxylin and eosin counter-
    stain is also recommended.
12. Dehydrate in 95% alcohol, then in absolute alcohol,
    two changes, 1 to 2 minutes each.
13. Clear in xylene, two changes.
14. Mount in Permount.

Results. Distinct outline of mesangial matrix, basement
          membrane of glomerulus: black. Nuclei: brown
          black. Hyaline: silver negative. Fibromucin:
          silver positive. Hyaline may be differentiated
          from overlaying epithelial cytoplasm by Masson's
          trichrome method in which hyaline stains green
          and cytoplasm rose. This method demonstrates
          the same structures as the periodic-acid-Schiff

technique but permits the resolution of delicate
structures unstained by the PAS method.

Note.   Glassware should be acid-cleaned and rinsed in
             distilled water.

Ref.   Jones, D. F., Nephrotic glomerulonephritis,
             Amer. J. Path., <u>33</u> (1957), 313-329.

MOWRY'S MODIFICATION OF THE HALE REACTION FOR ACID CARBOHYDRATE

<u>Fixation.</u>   10% buffered formalin, Helly's fluid.

SOLUTIONS

1.   Acetic acid solution.

     Glacial acetic acid   12 ml
     Distilled water   88 ml

2.   Ferric chloride, lumps U. S. P.   29 gm
     Distilled water   100 ml

     To 250 ml of boiling distilled water add 4.4 ml of
     29% ferric chloride solution and stir. When solution
     has turned red, remove from heat and allow to cool.
     The reagent is dark red, clear, and stable for many
     months. If the water is not kept boiling during the
     ferric chloride addition, the conversion to colloidal
     ferric oxide will be incomplete and results of its
     use will be faulty.

3.   Working solution of colloidal iron.

     Glacial acetic acid   5 ml
     Distilled water   15 ml
     Stock colloidal iron   20 ml

4.   Hydrochloric acid-potassium ferrocyanide solution.

     Hydrochloric acid   2% aqueous
     Potassium ferrocyanide   2% aqueous

     Mix equal parts just before use.

5.   Nuclear fast red (Kernechtrot)* counterstain.

Nuclear fast red   0.1 gm
Aluminum sulfate, 5% aqueous   100 ml

Dissolve the nuclear fast red in the aluminum sulfate solution with the aid of heat, cool, and filter.
Add crystal of thymol; keeps well at room temperature. Can be reused.

PROCEDURE

1.   Deparaffinize and hydrate sections. (Use control
     slide.)
2.   Remove mercury crystals if necessary.
3.   Rinse briefly in 12% acetic acid solution, 30 sec-
     onds.
4.   Place in freshly prepared working solution of col-
     loidal iron for 60 minutes. Do not place control
     slide in solution.
5.   Rinse in 4 changes of 12% acetic acid, 3 minutes
     each.
6.   Place sections, and control slide, in freshly pre-
     pared hydrochloric acid-potassium ferrocyanide re-
     agent for 20 minutes at room temperature.
7.   Wash gently in tap water for 5 minutes.
8.   Counterstain nuclei in Nuclear fast red for 5 min-
     utes.
9.   Rinse in tap water.
10. Dehydrate in 95% alcohol, then in absolute alcohol,
     two changes, 1 to 2 minutes each.
11. Clear in xylene, two changes.
12. Mount in Permount.

Results.   Sites of acid mucopolysaccharides: bright blue.
           Nuclei: red.

Ref.   Mowry, R.W., Lab. Invest., 7 (1958), 566-576.
           Copyright The Williams & Wilkins Co.

*Nuclear fast red (Kernechtrot), Roboz Surgical Instru-
  ment Co., Washington, D.C.

LENDRUM'S PICRO-MALLORY METHOD TO DEMONSTRATE FIBRIN

<u>Fixation</u>.   Formalin-mercuric chloride, Helly's fluid.

SOLUTIONS

1.   Celestin blue. Dissolve 5 gm of iron alum (ferric
      ammonium sulfate) overnight at room temperature in
      100 ml of distilled water. Bring to a boil and add
      0.5 gm of celestin blue and boil for 3 minutes.
      Cool, filter, and add 14 ml of glycerin. Solution
      lasts for months.

2.   Mayer's hemalum.

      Hematoxylin crystals   1 gm
      Sodium iodate   0.2 gm
      Aluminum and ammonium sulfate
      (ammonia alum)   50 gm
      Distilled water   1000 ml
      Chloral hydrate   50 gm
      Citric acid   1 gm

      Dissolve hematoxylin, sodium iodate, and the ammo-
      nia alum overnight in 1000 ml of distilled water.
      Add the chloral hydrate and citric acid. Boil for
      5 minutes; when cool, it is ready for use. The solu-
      tion keeps well.

3.   Picric acid-orange G solution.

      Saturated solution of picric acid
      in 80% alcohol (about 9%)   200 ml
      Orange G   0.4 gm
      Lissamine fast yellow 2G*   0.4 gm

4.   Acid fuchsin solution.

      Acid fuchsin   1 gm
      Distilled water   100 ml
      Glacial acetic acid   1 ml

5.   Differentiating solution.

      Stock picric acid-orange G (solution 3) 30 ml
      80% alcohol   70 ml

*Lissamine fast yellow 2G, ESBE Laboratory Supplies,
Toronto, Ontario, Canada.

6.	Phosphotungstic acid	1 gm
	Distilled water	100 ml

7.	Aniline blue	1 gm
	Distilled water	100 ml
	Glacial acetic acid	1 ml

PROCEDURE

1. Deparaffinize and hydrate sections.
2. Postmordant formalin-fixed tissue in a saturated aqueous mercuric chloride for 1 to 2 hours. (About 7.5 gm/100 ml).
3. Wash well in tap water.
4. Remove mercury crystals.
5. Stain in celestin blue for 10 minutes.
6. Wash in water.
7. Stain in Mayer's hemalum for 5 minutes.
8. Wash in tap water.
9. Check nuclei and differentiate in acid alcohol if necessary, then wash in tap water until blue.
10. Stain in picric acid-orange G stock solution for 3 to 5 minutes.
11. Wash in water for 1 minute.
12. Stain in acid fuchsin solution for 5 minutes.
13. Rinse in tap water.
14. Differentiate sections individually 3 to 5 seconds with microscopic control using a dropper bottle with solution 5. Do not overdifferentiate; the lissamine should replace the fuchsin in the red blood cells which take on a brilliant yellow color.
15. Rinse in tap water.
16. Place in phosphotungstic acid solution for 5 minutes, or longer if the collagen is dense.
17. Counterstain in aniline blue for 2 to 3 minutes.
18. Rinse in tap water.
19. Dehydrate in 95% alcohol for 1 minute.
20. Dehydrate in absolute alcohol, two changes, 1 to 2 minutes each.
21. Clear in xylene, two changes.
22. Mount in Permount.

Results. Nuclei: blue-black. Cytoplasm: mauve. Chromatin: dark purple. Collagen and reticulin: blue. Elastic fibers: dull red. Fibrin: brilliant red. Red blood cells: brilliant yellow. Muscle: dull red.

Note. Reasonably well formalin fixed tissue briefly followed by mercuric chloride post-mordanting

shows pale yellow erythrocytes. In tissue
otherwise or poorly fixed erythrocytes tend to
retain the red of the acid fuchsin, instead of
being brilliant yellow.

Ref.   Personal communication.

PUTT'S MODIFICATION OF THE M. S. B. METHOD TO
DEMONSTRATE FIBRIN

Fixation.   Helly's fluid. Postmordant formalin-fixed
              material in a saturated aqueous solution of
              mercuric chloride for 1 hour.

SOLUTIONS

1.   Lendrum's celestin blue.

      Dissolve 5 gm of iron alum (ferric ammonium sulfate)
      overnight at room temperature in 100 ml of distilled
      water. Bring to a boil, add 0.5 gm of celestin blue,
      and boil for 3 minutes. Filter when cool and add 14
      ml of glycerin. Solution keeps for months.

2.   Mayer's hemalum.

      Hematoxylin crystals   1 gm
      Sodium iodate   0.2 gm
      Aluminum and ammonium sulfate
      (ammonia alum)   50 gm
      Distilled water   1000 ml
      Chloral hydrate   50 gm
      Citric acid   1 gm

      Dissolve the hematoxylin, sodium iodate, and ammo-
      nia alum overnight in the distilled water. Add
      chloral hydrate and citric acid and boil for 5 min-
      utes. When cool, it is ready for use. This solu-
      tion keeps well for 2 to 3 months.

3.   Dissolve 0.5 gm of martius yellow in 20 ml of dis-
      tilled water and 2 gm of phosphomolybdic acid in 80
      ml of absolute alcohol. Combine solutions.

4.   Fast fuchsin 6B solution.*

    Fast fuchsin 6B (C. I. No. 16600)   1 gm
    Glacial acetic acid   2 ml
    Distilled water   98 ml

5.   Methyl blue solution.

    Methyl blue   0.5 gm
    Glacial acetic acid   2 ml
    Distilled water   98 ml

6.   1% aqueous glacial acetic acid.

PROCEDURE

1.   Deparaffinize and hydrate sections.
2.   Postmordant formalin-fixed material.
3.   Remove mercury crystals.
4.   Stain in celestin blue for 5 minutes.
5.   Wash in water.
6.   Stain in Mayer's hemalum for 5 minutes.
7.   Wash well in water.
8.   If necessary differentiate in acid alcohol (1 ml
     hydrochloric acid in 99 ml of 70% alcohol).
9.   Wash well in running tap water.
10. Rinse in 80% alcohol.
11. Stain in martius yellow for 3 to 5 minutes.
12. Rinse in 80% alcohol.
13. Rinse in distilled water.
14. Stain in fast fuchsin for 10 to 15 minutes. (Check
     staining of fibrin under microscope.)
15. Rinse in two changes of distilled water.
16. Counterstain in methyl blue for 30 seconds to 1
     minute.
17. Rinse in distilled water.
18. Place in 1% acetic acid for 3 to 4 minutes.
19. Dehydrate in 95% alcohol, then in absolute alcohol,
     two changes, 1 to 2 minutes each.
20. Clear in xylene, two changes.
21. Mount in Permount.

Results.   Nuclei: blue-black. Erythrocytes: yellow.
           Fibrin: red. Connective tissue: blue.
Ref.   Unpublished.

*Fast fuchsin 6B, Allied Chemicals, National Aniline
Division (C. I. No. 16600), acid violet 6. This modification permits the use of domestic dyes.

SLIDDER'S FRASER'S, AND LENDRUM'S M. S. B. METHOD TO
DEMONSTRATE FIBRIN

<u>Fixation</u>.   Formol-sublimate or formol-saline or Helly's
           fluid. Formol-saline-fixed material is placed
           in 5% aqueous mercuric chloride for 2 to 3
           weeks.

SOLUTIONS

1.   Lendrum's celestin blue.

      Dissolve 5 gm of iron alum (ferric ammonium sulfate)
      overnight at room temperature in 100 ml of distilled
      water. Bring to a boil and add 0.5 gm of celestin
      blue and boil for 3 minutes. Filter when cool and
      add 14 ml of glycerine. Solution keeps for months.

2.   Mayer's hemalum.

Hematoxylin crystals	1 gm
Sodium iodate	0.2 gm
Aluminum and ammonium sulfate (ammonia alum)	50 gm
Distilled water	1000 ml
Chloral hydrate	50 gm
Citric acid	1 gm

      Dissolve the hematoxylin, sodium iodate and ammonia
      alum overnight in the distilled water. Add chloral
      hydrate and citric acid and boil for 5 minutes.
      When cool it is ready for use. This solution keeps
      well for 2 to 3 months.

3.   Acid alcohol.

70% alcohol	99 ml
Hydrochloric acid	1 ml

4.   Martius yellow solution.

Martius yellow	0.5 gm
95% alcohol	100 ml
Phosphotungstic acid	2 gm

5.   Brilliant crystal scarlet 6R solution.*

Brilliant crystal scarlet 6R   2.5 gm
Glacial acetic acid   2.5 ml
Distilled water   98 ml

6.   1% aqueous phosphomolybdic acid.

7.   Soluble blue solution.[†]

Soluble blue   0.5 gm
Glacial acetic acid   1 ml
Distilled water   98 ml

PROCEDURE

 1.   Deparaffinize and hydrate sections.
 2.   Remove mercury crystals.
 3.   Stain in celestin blue for 5 minutes.
 4.   Wash in water.
 5.   Stain in Mayer's hemalum for 5 minutes.
 6.   Wash in tap water.
 7.   Differentiate briefly in acid alcohol.
 8.   Wash well in running tap water until nuclei are blue.
 9.   Rinse in 95% alcohol.
10.   Stain in martius yellow for 2 minutes.
11.   Rinse in distilled water.
12.   Stain in brilliant crystal scarlet for 10 minutes.
13.   Rinse in distilled water.
14.   Place in phosphotungstic acid solution for 5 minutes.
15.   Rinse in distilled water.
16.   Stain in soluble blue for 10 minutes.
17.   Rinse in water, blot slide with filter paper.
18.   Rinse slide with absolute alcohol from dropper
       bottle.
19.   Clear in xylene, two changes.
20.   Mount in Permount.

Results.   Fibrin: red. Nuclie: blue-black. Erythro-
            cytes: yellow. Connective tissue: blue.

Ref.   Lendrum, A. C., Fraser, D. S., Slidders, W.,
            and Henderson, R., J. Clin. Path., 15 (1962),
            401-413.

*Brilliant crystal scarlet, L. B. Holliday Lt. Dyeworks,
Huddersfield.
† Soluble blue-Aniline blue (C. I. No. 42755), Allied
Chemicals, National Aniline Division.

WEIGERT'S METHOD TO DEMONSTRATE FIBRIN

Fixation.   10% formalin, absolute alcohol, Zenker or
            Helly's fluid.

SOLUTIONS

1. Aqueous crystal violet.

    Crystal violet   1 gm
    Distilled water   100 ml

2. Gram's iodine.

    Iodine crystals   1 gm
    Potassium iodide   2 gm
    Distilled water   300 ml

    Dissolve the potassium iodide in a small amount of
    water. Add the iodine crystals. When dissolved,
    add the balance of the water.

3. Aniline-xylene 50/50.   Shake well.

4. Neutral red solution.

    Neutral red   1 gm
    Distilled water   100 ml

PROCEDURE

1. Deparaffinize and hydrate sections.
2. Place sections on staining rack and pour on crystal
    violet solution; allow to act for 3 minutes. Filter
    before use.
3. Rinse in tap water.
4. Treat with Gram's iodine for 3 minutes.
5. Blot dry with filter paper.
6. Decolorize with aniline-xylene from a dropper bottle
    until the fibrin is blue and background nearly color-
    less. (Control with microscope.)
7. Rinse in xylene to remove aniline and blot dry.
8. Stain in neutral red for 1 to 2 minutes.
9. Rinse rapidly in distilled water. Blot dry and dif-
    ferentiate neutral red in aniline. (Control with
    microscope.)
10. Clear in xylene, two changes.
11. Mount in Permount.

Results.   Fibrin: blue. Gram-positive bacteria: blue-black. Other tissue elements: shades of red.

Ref.   Mallory, F. B., Pathological Technique, Hafner Publishing Co., New York 1968.

BEST'S CARMINE METHOD TO DEMONSTRATE GLYCOGEN

Fixation. Rossman's, Carnoy's, 10% formalin, Helly's fluid. Absolute alcohol is not recommended, as it causes polarization of glycogen.

SOLUTIONS

1.   Harris' hematoxylin.

Hematoxylin crystals	5 gm
Absolute ethyl alcohol	50 ml
Aluminum and potassium sulfate (potassium alum)	100 gm
Mercuric oxide (red)	2.5 gm
Distilled water	1000 ml

Dissolve the hematoxylin in the alcohol and the alum in water with the aid of heat. Mix the two solutions together and bring to a boil. Withdraw the flame; slowly and carefully add the mercuric oxide. Heat gently and allow to boil for 5 minutes. Place the flask in cold water and cool quickly. Filter and add 40 ml of glacial acetic acid to improve nuclear staining. Filter the solution each time before use. Solution effective for 1 to 2 months.

2.   Best's carmine stock solution.

Carmine alum lake (C. I. No. 75470)	2 gm
Potassium carbonate	1 gm
Potassium chloride	5 gm
Distilled water	60 ml
Ammonium hydroxide 28%	20 ml

Boil gently and cautiously for several minutes. After cooling add the ammonium hydroxide. Keep stock solution in refrigerator in a dark bottle. Solution keeps for 5 to 6 weeks.

3.   Best's carmine working solution.

Stock carmine solution, freshly
filtered   10 ml
Ammonium hydroxide 28%   15 ml
Methyl alcohol   15 ml

Discard after use.

4.   Best's differentiator.

Methyl alcohol   40 ml
Ethyl alcohol   80 ml
Distilled water   100 ml

PROCEDURE

1.   Deparaffinize sections to absolute alcohol.
2.   Stain in Harris' hematoxylin for 5 minutes.
3.   Wash in tap water; differentiate in acid alcohol if
     necessary.
4.   Rinse in water, bluing in tap water is unnecessary.
     The ammonia in the staining solution will accomplish
     this.
5.   Place in Best's working solution for 5 to 10 minutes.
6.   Differentiate in Best's differentiator until clouds
     of stain no longer come off. (Three changes of abso-
     lute methyl alcohol may be substituted in place of
     Best's differentiator.)
7.   If Best's differentiator is used, pass slides
     through three changes of absolute alcohol. (If
     methyl alcohol is used pass slides through two
     changes of acetone.)
8.   Clear in xylene, two changes.
9.   Mount in Permount.

Results.   Glycogen: red. Nuclei: blue. This method also
           stains the corpora amylacea of the central ner-
           vous system.

Ref.   Best, F., Z. Wiss. Mikroskop., 23 (1906) 319.
           Mallory, F. B., Pathological Technique, Hafner
           Publishing Co., New York, 1968.

THE BAUER REACTION FOR GLYCOGEN

Fixation.   Cold 10% buffered formalin, Rossman's or
            Helly's fluid.

SOLUTIONS

1.   Chromic acid.

     Chromic acid   4 gm
     Distilled water   100 ml

2.   Normal hydrochloric acid.

     Hydrochloric acid, sp. gr. 1.19   83.5 ml
     Distilled water   916.5 ml

3.   Schiff reagent. Bring 200 ml of distilled water to
     a boil, remove from flame, add 1 gm of basic fuchsin,
     and stir until dissolved. Cool to 50°C. Filter and
     add 20 ml of normal hydrochloric acid. Cool further
     to 25°C. Add 1 gm of sodium or potassium metabisul-
     fite, (Na2S205, K2S205), place in the dark in a
     stoppered bottle for 18 to 24 hours; solution takes
     on an orange color. Add 0.5 gm of activated char-
     coal and shake well, then filter through a coarse
     filter paper. Store under refrigeration in a brown
     stoppered bottle of the same volume. Solution is
     stable for several weeks. Use at room temperature.

4.   Sulfurous acid rinse.

     10% sodium metabisulfite   6 ml
     Normal hydrochloric acid   5 ml
     Distilled water   100 ml

5.   Harris' hematoxylin.

     Hematoxylin crystals   5 gm
     Absolute ethyl alcohol   50 ml
     Aluminum and potassium sulfate
     (potassium alum)   100 gm
     Mercuric oxide (red)   2.5 gm
     Distilled water   1000 ml

     Dissolve the hematoxylin in the alcohol and the alum
     in water with the aid of heat. Mix the two solutions
     together and bring to a boil. Withdraw the flame,
     slowly and carefully add the mercuric oxide, heat
     gently, and allow to boil for 5 minutes. Place the

flask in cold water and cool quickly. Filter and add 40 ml of glacial acetic acid to improve nuclear staining. Filter the solution each time before use, solution effective for 1 to 2 months.

PROCEDURE

1. Deparaffinize and hydrate sections. (Use control slide.)
2. Rinse in distilled water.
3. Place in freshly prepared chromic acid for 1 hour.
4. Wash in running tap water for 5 minutes.
5. Place in Schiff solution for 15 minutes.
6. Rinse in three changes of sulfurous acid rinse for 2 minutes each. Discard solution.
7. Wash in running tap water for 10 minutes.
8. Stain nuclei in Harris' hematoxylin for 2 minutes.
9. Wash well in tap water.
10. Dehydrate in 95% alcohol and absolute alcohol, two changes, 1 to 2 minutes each.
11. Clear in xylene, two changes.
12. Mount in Permount.

Results.   Glycogen: red or reddish purple. Nuclei: blue.

Ref.   McManus, J. F. A. and Mowry, R. W., Staining Methods Histologic and Histochemical, Harper & Row, New York, 1963.

HIGHMAN'S CONGO RED METHOD TO DEMONSTRATE AMYLOID

Fixation. 10% formalin.

SOLUTIONS

1. Congo red.

   Congo red   0.5 gm
   50% alcohol   100 ml

2. Potassium hydroxide.

   Potassium hydroxide   0.2 gm
   80% alcohol   100 ml

3. Mayer's hemalum.

Hematoxylin crystals	1 gm
Sodium iodate	0.2 gm
Aluminum and ammonium sulfate (ammonia alum)	50 ml
Distilled water	1000 ml
Chloral hydrate	50 gm
Citric acid	1 gm

Dissolve hematoxylin, sodium iodate, and the ammonia alum overnight in 1000 ml of distilled water. Add the chloral hydrate and citric acid. Boil for 5 minutes; when cool, it is ready for use. The solution keeps well.

PROCEDURE

1. Deparaffinize and hydrate sections to 50% alcohol. (Run control slide.)
2. Stain in Highman's Congo red for 5 minutes.
3. Differentiate in potassium hydroxide for 1 to 3 minutes. (Discard).
4. Rinse in tap water.
5. Stain nuclei in Mayer's hemalum for 2 to 3 minutes.
6. Wash in running tap water for 5 minutes.
7. Dehydrate in 95% alcohol then absolute alcohol, two changes, 1 to 2 minutes each.
8. Clear in xylene, two changes.
9. Mount in Permount.

Results. Amyloid: red. Nuclei: Blue.

Note. Congo red and acid fuchsin are very alkaline sensitive and are not safe after hematoxylin stains which have been blued in alkaline solutions. Precut control slides for all of the amyloid stains are effective for about 6 months.

Ref. Highman, B. AMA., Arch. Path., 41 (1946), 559-562. Copyright American Medical Association

BENNHOLD'S CONGO RED METHOD FOR AMYLOID

Fixation. Absolute alcohol or 10% formalin.

SOLUTIONS

1. Congo red solution.

| Congo red | 1 gm |
| Distilled water | 100 ml |

2.   Saturated aqueous solution of lithium carbonate (2 gm per 100 ml).

3.   80% alcohol.

4.   Harris' hematoxylin.

Hematoxylin crystals	5 gm
Absolute ethyl alcohol	50 ml
Aluminum and potassium sulfate (potassium alum)	100 gm
Mercuric oxide (red)	2.5 gm
Distilled water	1000 ml

Dissolve the hematoxylin in the alcohol and the alum in water with the aid of heat. Mix the two solutions together and bring to a boil. Withdraw the flame; slowly and carefully add the mercuric oxide. Heat gently and allow to continue to boil for 5 minutes. Place the flask in cold water and cool quickly. Filter and add 40 ml of glacial acetic acid to improve nuclear staining. Filter the solution each time before use. Solution effective for 1 to 2 months.

PROCEDURE

1.   Deparaffinize and hydrate sections. (Run control slide.)
2.   Stain in Congo red solution for 10 to 20 minutes.
3.   Dip in saturated lithium carbonate for 15 seconds. (Discard.)
4.   Rinse in 80% alcohol until excess dye disappears. (Discard.)
5.   Wash in running tap water for 15 minutes.
6.   Counterstain in Harris' hematoxylin for 2 to 3 minutes.
7.   Wash well in running tap water.
8.   Dehydrate in 95% alcohol, then in absolute alcohol, two changes, 1 to 2 minutes each.
9.   Clear in xylene, two changes.
10. Mount in Permount.

Results.   Amyloid: red.   Nuclei: blue.   At times other hyaline material may be colored red.

Note.   The procedure may be reversed, with the nuclear
             staining preceding the Congo red.

Ref.   Bennhold, H., Munch. Med. Woch., 1922, pp.
             1537-1538.

PUCHTLER, SWEAT, AND LEVINE'S CONGO RED METHOD TO
DEMONSTRATE AMYLOID

Fixation.   Carnoy's fluid, absolute alcohol, 10% formalin,
             Helly's fluid.

SOLUTIONS

  1. Mayer's hemalum.

      Hematoxylin crystals   1 gm
      Sodium iodate   0.2 gm

      Aluminum and ammonium sulfate
      (ammonia alum)   50 gm
      Distilled water   1000 ml
      Chloral hydrate   50 gm
      Citric acid   1 gm

      Dissolve hematoxylin, sodium iodate, and the ammo-
      nia alum overnight in 1000 ml of distilled water.
      Add chloral hydrate and citric acid. Boil for 5
      minutes; when cool, it is ready for use. This solu-
      tion keeps well.

  2. Stock alkaline solution.

      80% ethyl alcohol saturated with sodium chloride
      1% aqueous sodium hydroxide

      Working solution. Mix fresh and use within 15 min-
      utes.

      1% aqueous sodium hydroxide   0.5 ml
      Saturated sodium chloride in ethyl
      alcohol   50 ml

  3. Congo red solution (Harleco).

      80% ethyl alcohol saturated with Congo red (2 gm)
      and sodium chloride; allow to stand for 24 hours.

      Working solution. Filter; use within 15 minutes.

1% aqueous sodium hydroxide	0.5 ml
Saturated Congo red solution	50 ml

PROCEDURE

1. Deparaffinize and hydrate sections. (Run control slide.)
2. Remove mercury crystals if necessary.
3. Stain in Mayer's hemalum for 10 minutes.
4. Rinse in three changes of distilled water.
5. Alkalize in solution 2 for 20 minutes.
6. Stain in Congo red solution for 20 minutes.
7. Dehydrate rapidly in three changes of absolute alcohol.
8. Clear in xylene, two changes.
9. Mount in Permount.

Results.   Amyloid: deep pink to red. Nuclei: blue. Background: yellow.

Ref.   Puchtler, H., Sweat, F., and Levine, J., J. Histochem. Cytochem., 10 (1962), 355-364. Copyright the Williams, Wilkins Co.

LIEB CRYSTAL VIOLET METHOD TO DEMONSTRATE AMYLOID

Fixation.   10% formalin.

SOLUTIONS

1. Crystal violet (stock solution).

Crystal violet (to saturate)	14 gm
95% alcohol	100 ml

2. Crystal violet (working solution).

Crystal violet (stock solution)	10 ml
Distilled water	300 ml
Hydrochloric acid	1 ml

3. Valnor mounting media.*

Valnor	50 gm
Distilled water	25 ml

*Valnor mounting media, formerly called Abopon, Valnor Corporation, Brooklyn, N. Y.

PROCEDURE

1. Deparaffinize and hydrate sections. (Run control slide.)
2. Rinse in distilled water.
3. Stain in working solution of crystal violet for 1 to 2 minutes.
4. Rinse well in tap water.
5. Mount in Valnor.

Results.   Amyloid: purplish violet. Other tissue elements: blue.

Note.   Check staining under microscope without a blue glass filter. Amyloid preparations fade in a short time and should be examined or photographed as soon as possible if permanent records are to be kept.

            Unfixed tissue sectioned on the cryostat is by far the best procedure to demonstrate amyloid.

            The slides must be air-dried; do not use any type of fixative. Stain with Lieb's or Lillie's crystal violet procedure and mount in glycerin jelly prepared without the addition of carbolic acid. When dry, finished slides may be ringed with clear nail polish. Examine without blue filter on microscope.

Ref.   Lieb, E., Amer. J. Clin. Path., 17 (1947), 413-414.

CRYSTAL VIOLET METHOD TO DEMONSTRATE AMYLOID

Fixation.   10% formalin.

SOLUTIONS

1. 1% aqueous solution of crystal violet.

2. Lillie's modification.

Crystal violet	1 gm
Methyl violet 2B	0.5 gm
Absolute alcohol	10 ml
Distilled water	90 ml

3.   1% aqueous acetic acid.

4.   Baker's glycerin jelly.

Fine gelatin	5 gm
Cold distilled water	25 ml
Glycerin	35 ml
Distilled water	40 ml
Cresol	25 ml

Soak gelatin in distilled water for 1 hour. Cover
the vessel and place in paraffin oven. Stir from
time to time until the gelatin has dissolved. Mix
glycerin, water, and cresol. Place this mixture also
in the paraffin oven. When the gelatin has dissolved,
mix the solutions thoroughly and filter through folded gauze while still hot in the incubator. Will gel
when cool. For use, melt in incubator or in water
bath.

PROCEDURE

1.   Frozen or paraffin sections may be used. (Run con-
      trol slide.)
2.   Deparaffinize and hydrate paraffin sections.
3.   Place in crystal violet solution or Lillie's modifi-
      cation for 3 to 5 minutes.
4.   Wash in 1% acetic acid for 1 minute. (Discard.)
5.   Wash well in distilled water to remove all traces of
      acid.
6.   Mount directly in Baker's media or Lieb's Valnor
      media.

Results.   Amyloid and fibrinoid: violet. Other elements:
            blue.

Note.   Examine without blue filter on microscope.

LENDRUM'S DEHLIA METHOD TO DEMONSTRATE AMYLOID

Fixation.   10% formalin or absolute alcohol.

SOLUTIONS

1.   1% aqueous dahlia (methyl violet 2B C. I. No. 42535).

2.   Formalin differentiator.

      40% formaldehyde   70 ml
      Distilled water   30 ml

3.   Saturated aqueous solution of sodium chloride (about
      35 gm per 100 ml).

PROCEDURE

1.   Deparaffinize and hydrate sections. (Run control
      slide.)
2.   Stain in dahlia for 3 minutes.
3.   Differentiate in formalin solution. (Discard.)
4.   Rinse well in water.
5.   Place in sodium chloride solution for 5 minutes.
      (Discard.)
6.   Rinse well in water.
7.   Mount in Baker's or Lieb's Valnor media.

Results.   Amyloid: pink to red. Other structures: blue
            or violet.

Note.   This method gives preparations that remain
            stable for a number of years. Examine without
            blue filter on microscope.

Ref.   Lendrum, A. C., Recent Advances in Pathology,
            2nd ed., J. & A. Churchill, London, 1951.

MALLORY'S HEMATOXYLIN-PHLOXINE METHOD TO
DEMONSTRATE ALCOHOLIC HYALIN

Fixation.   10% formalin or absolute alcohol.

SOLUTIONS

1.   Mallory's alum hematoxylin.

      Hematoxylin   1 gm
      Aluminum or potassium alum   20 gm
      Distilled water   400 ml
      Thymol   1 gm

      Dissolve the hematoxylin in 100 ml of distilled
      water with the aid of heat. Add the alum dissolved
      in the rest of the water. When cool, add the thymol
      to prevent the growth of mold. Expose the solution
      to light and air in a lightly stoppered flask (cotton

plug). The solution will ripen in about 10 days,
after which it should be kept in a tightly stoppered
bottle. The solution lasts for 2 to 3 months.

2. Phloxine B solution.

Phloxine B	0.5 gm
20% alcohol	100 ml

3. Lithium carbonate solution.

Lithium carbonate	0.1 gm
Distilled water	100 ml

PROCEDURE

1. Deparaffinize and hydrate sections.
2. Stain in Mallory's alum hematoxylin for 4 to 5 min-
    utes.
3. Wash well in running tap water until the section is
    blue.
4. Stain in phloxine B for 20 to 60 minutes.
5. Wash in tap water.
6. Decolorize in lithium carbonate for 30 to 60 seconds.
    (Discard.)
7. Wash in tap water.
8. Dehydrate in 95% alcohol then absolute alcohol, two
    changes, 1 to 2 minutes each.
9. Clear in xylene, two changes.
10. Mount in Permount.

Results.   Nuclei: blue. Fresh hyalin appears as red
             droplets and threads. Older hyalin: pink to
             colorless.

Ref.   Mallory, F. B., Pathological Technique, Hafner
             Publishing Co., New York, 1968.

JANSCO'S CHLORAZOL FAST PINK METHOD FOR
POLYVINYL PYRROLIDONE (PVP)

Fixation. 10% formalin.

SOLUTIONS

1. Chlorazol fast pink.*

*Chlorazol fast pink, National Aniline Division, Allied
 Chemical Corporation.

| 50% ethyl alcohol | 100 ml |
| Chlorazol fast pink | 1 gm |

2. Mayer's hemalum.

Hematoxylin crystals	1 gm
Sodium iodate	0.2 gm
Aluminum and ammonium sulfate	
(ammonia alum)	50 gm
Distilled water	1000 ml
Chloral hydrate	50 gm
Citric acid	1 gm

Dissolve hematoxylin, sodium iodate, and the ammonia alum overnight in 1000 ml of distilled water.
Add the chloral hydrate and citric acid. Boil for
5 minutes; when cool, it is ready for use. The
solution keeps well.

3. Acid alcohol.

| 70% alcohol | 99 ml |
| Hydrochloric acid | 1 ml |

PROCEDURE

1. Deparaffinize and hydrate sections.
2. Stain in chlorazol fast pink for 10 to 30 minutes
    in 60°C oven, in covered Coplin jar.
3. Rinse in water.
4. Stain nuclei in Mayer's hemalum for 3 minutes.
5. Wash in tap water.
6. Differentiate in acid alcohol.
7. Wash in tap water until nuclei are blue.
8. Dehydrate in 95% alcohol, then in absolute alcohol,
    two changes, 1 to 2 minutes each.
9. Clear in xylene.
10. Mount in Permount.

Results. PVP stains pink to cherry red. Nuclei: blue.

Ref.   Pearse, A. G. E., Histochemistry Theoretical
          and Applied, 2nd ed., Little, Brown, Boston,
          1960.

FONTANA-MASSON METHOD TO DEMONSTRATE ARGENTAFFIN GRANULES

Fixation. To demonstrate argentaffin cells (also called enterochromaffin or Kultchitsky cells) tissue must be fixed immediately in 10% formalin or preferably formol-saline. Alcohol or fixatives containing corrosive sublimate or acetic acid must be avoided. These granules can rarely be demonstrated in autopsy material.

SOLUTIONS

1. Fontana's silver solution. In a chemically clean flask make up a 5% aqueous solution of silver nitrate, add carefully drop by drop 28% ammonium hydroxide until the precipitate formed is exactly redissolved; then carefully add 5% aqueous solution of silver nitrate drop by drop until the appearance of a persistent cloudiness does not disappear on shaking. This solution should not smell of ammonia. Let stand overnight before using; filter before use. Solution is good for several months. Lillie prefers to prepare a small quantity fresh each time.

2. Toning solution.

    1:500 aqueous yellow gold chloride

3. Sodium thiosulfate (hypo)   5 gm
    Distilled water   100 ml

4. Counterstain.

    Neutral red   1 gm
    Distilled water   99 ml
    Glacial acetic acid   1 ml

PROCEDURE

1. Deparaffinize and hydrate sections.
2. Wash well in distilled water.
3. Place sections in Fontana's silver solution in the dark at room temperature for 36 to 40 hours in covered Coplin jar.
4. Wash in many changes of distilled water.
5. Tone in gold chloride for 5 minutes.
6. Wash in distilled water.
7. Fix in sodium thiosulfate for 5 minutes.
8. Rinse in distilled water.
9. Counterstain in Neutral red for 1 minute if desired.
10. Rinse in 95% alcohol, then absolute alcohol, two changes, 1 to 2 minutes each.

11.   Mount in Permount.

Results.   Argentaffin granules: black. Other tissue ele-
            ments: depend on the counterstain.

Ref.   Masson, P., Amer. J. Path., _4_ (1928), 181-212.

BURTNER-LILLIE METHENAMINE SILVER METHOD FOR
ARGENTAFFIN GRANULES

Fixation. Formol-saline or 10% formalin. Alcohol or alco-
           hol-containing fixatives should not be used;
           argentaffin granules are soluble in alcohol.

SOLUTIONS

1.   Weigert's iodine.

      Iodine crystals   1 gm
      Potassium iodide   2 gm
      Distilled water   100 ml

      Dissolve the potassium iodide in a small amount of
      water. Add the iodine. When dissolved, add the
      balance of the water.

2.   Sodium thiosulfate   5 gm
      Distilled water   100 ml

3.   Stock methenamine silver solution.

      Methenamine 3% aqueous   100 ml
      Silver nitrate 5% aqueous   5 ml

      A white precipitate appears but dissolves immediately
      on shaking. The clear solution lasts for months if
      kept refrigerated.

4.   Holmes' borate buffer solution.

      0.2M boric acid   12.4 gm per 1000 ml
      0.05M borax   19.0 gm per 1000 ml

      pH 7.8   0.2M boric acid 16 ml   0.05M borax 4 ml

5.   Methenamine silver working solution.

| Stock silver solution | 30 ml |
| Borate buffer pH 7.8 | 8 ml |

6. Toning solution.

    1:500 aqueous yellow gold chloride

| 7. Sodium thiosulfate | 5 gm |
| Distilled water | 100 ml |

8. Safranin counterstain.

Safranin O	1 gm
Distilled water	100 ml
Add a few drops of glacial acetic acid.	

PROCEDURE

1. Deparaffinize and hydrate sections.
2. Place in Weigert's iodine for 10 minutes.
3. Bleach in sodium thiosulfate for 2 minutes.
4. Wash in running tap water for 10 minutes.
5. Rinse in two changes of distilled water.
6. Place section in Coplin jar containing preheated buffered methenamine silver solution and put in 60°C oven for 2 to 3 hours.
7. Rinse in distilled water.
8. Tone in gold chloride solution for 10 minutes.
9. Rinse in distilled water.
10. Fix in sodium thiosulfate solution for 2 minutes.
11. Wash in running tap water for 5 minutes.
12. Counterstain in safranin for 5 minutes.
13. Dehydrate in acetone.
14. Clear in xylene, two changes.
15. Mount in Permount.

Results. Argentaffin granules: black. Nucelei: red.

Note.   All glassware should be acid-cleaned and rinsed in distilled water.

Ref.   Burtner, H. J. and Lillie, R. D., Stain Tech., 24 (1949), 225-227. Copyright the Williams and Wilkins Co.

MODIFIED METHOD TO DEMONSTRATE ENTEROCHROME GRANULES

Fixation. 10% formalin.

SOLUTIONS

1.   Ferric-ferricyanide solution.

       Potassium ferricyanide, 1% aqueous   10 ml
       Ferric chloride, 1% aqueous   75 ml
       Distilled water   15 ml

2.   Safranin O (C. I. No. 50240) counterstain.

       Safranin O   1 gm
       20% alcohol   100 ml

PROCEDURE

1.   Deparaffinize and hydrate sections.
2.   Rinse in distilled water.
3.   Stain in freshly prepared ferric-ferricyanide for 5
4.   minutes.
     Rinse in three changes of distilled water.
5.   Counterstain in safranin solution for 2 to 5 minutes.
6.   Rinse in tap water.
7.   Dehydrate in 95% alcohol, then in absolute alcohol,
     two changes, 1 to 2 minutes each.
8.   Clear in xylene.
9.   Mount in Permount.

Results.   Enterochromaffin granules: blue. Nuclei: red.

Ref.   Lillie R. D., Histopatholigical Technic and
            Practical Histo-Chemistry, used with permis-
            sion of McGraw-Hill, 3rd ed., New York, 1965.

DIAZONIUM REACTION TO DEMONSTRATE ENTEROCHROME GRANULES

Fixation.   10% formalin.

SOLUTIONS

1.   Garnet salt GBC.*

     Garnet salt GBC   0.5 gm

*Garnet salt GBC, ESBE Laboratory Supplies, Toronto,
Ontario, Canada.

Distilled water	100 ml
Saturated aqueous solution of borax (about 6 gm per 100 ml)	2.5 ml

2.   Mayer's hemalum.

Hematoxylin crystals	1 gm
Sodium iodate	0.2 gm
Aluminum and ammonium sulfate (ammonia alum)	50 gm
Distilled water	1000 ml
Chloral hydrate	50 gm
Citric acid	1 gm

Dissolve hematoxylin, sodium iodate, and the ammonia alum overnight in 1000 ml of distilled water. Add the chloral hydrate and citric acid. Boil for 5 minutes; when cool, it is ready for use. The solution keeps well.

PROCEDURE

1.   Deparaffinize and hydrate sections.
2.   Rinse in distilled water.
3.   Stain in Garnet solution for 30 to 60 seconds.
4.   Wash in running tap water for 30 seconds.
5.   Stain nuclei in Mayer's hemalum for 2 to 3 minutes.
6.   Wash in running tap water for 5 minutes.
7.   Dehydrate in 95% alcohol, then in absolute alcohol, two changes, 1 to 2 minutes each.
8.   Clear in xylene, two changes.
9.   Mount in Permount.

Results.   Enterochrome granules: red. Nuclei: blue. Background: yellow.

Ref.   McManus, J. F. A. and Mowry, R. W., Staining Methods Histologic and Histochemical, Harper & Row, New York, 1963.

MODIFIED SCHMORL'S METHOD TO DEMONSTRATE ADRENOCHROME

Fixation.

3% aqueous potassium dichromate	80 ml
Formaldehyde 40%	20 ml

Fix tissue for 24 hours; wash for 1 to 2 hours in running tap water.

SOLUTIONS

1.   Stock Giemsa solution*
        Distilled water

        Add 1 drop of Giemsa stain to each ml of
        distilled water.

PROCEDURE

1.   Deparaffinize and hydrate sections.
2.   Stain sections for 15 to 24 hours in dilute Giemsa
        stain.
3.   Rinse in tap water, then in distilled water.
4.   Blot dry with fine filter paper.
5.   Dehydrate rapidly with acetone.
6.   Pass rapidly through equal parts of acetone-xylene.
7.   Clear in xylene.
8.   Mount in Permount

Results.   Medullary cells: bright red to violet. Corti-
            cal cells: blue. Erythrocytes: pink. Eosino-
            phil granules: red.

Ref.   McManus, J. F. A. and Mowry, R. W., Staining
            Methods Histologic and Histochemical, Harper &
            Row, New York, 1963.

BUNTING'S MOLYBDATE REACTION FOR PHOSPHATES

Fixation.   10% formalin.

SOLUTIONS

1. a. Ammonium molybdate   5 gm
        Distilled water   100 ml

    b. Nitric acid   1 ml
        Distilled water   99 ml

    Use in equal parts.

2. Benzidine solution.

    Benzidine base[†]   50 mg
    Glacial acetic acid   10 ml

*Stock Giemsa, Gradwold Laboratories, St. Louis, Mo.
[†]Benzidine base, Hartman-Leddon Co., Philadelphia, Pa.

3.   Saturated aqueous sodium acetate (about 45%).

PROCEDURE

1.   Deparaffinize and hydrate to distilled water.
2.   Cover section with ammonium molybdate-nitric acid
      solution for 5 minutes.
3.   Wash well in distilled water.
4.   Cover with benzidine solution for 1 minute.
5.   Flood with sodium acetate solution, apply cover
      glass, and examine at once.

Results.   Areas of phosphate ion: blue. The color fades
            in a few hours.

Ref.   Personal communication.

HALL'S METHOD TO DEMONSTRATE BILIRUBIN

Fixation.   10% formalin, Bouin's, or Carnoy's fluid.
            Helly and Zenker fluids are unsuitable.

SOLUTIONS

1.   Fouchet's reagent.

      Trichloracetic acid   25 gm
      Distilled water   100 ml
      Ferric chloride (10% aqueous)   10 ml

2.   Van Gieson's counterstain.

      Solution A   Solution B
      Acid fuchsin   1 gm   Saturated aqueous solution
      Saturated aqueous   of picric acid
      solution of picric
      acid   100 ml

      To use, combine 1 ml of solution A with 10 ml of
      solution B.

PROCEDURE

1.   Deparaffinize and hydrate sections.
2.   Stain in Fouchet's reagent for 5 minutes.
3   Wash well in tap water.
4.   Counterstain in Van Gieson's picro-fuchsin for 5
      minutes.

5.   Differentiate in 95% alcohol, 30 seconds.
6.   Dehydrate in absolute alcohol, two changes, 1 to 2
     minutes each.
7.   Clear in xylene, two changes.
8.   Mount in Permount.

Results.   Bilirubin oxidized to biliverdin, olive green
           to emerald green, depending on concentration
           of biliverdin.

Ref.   Hall, M. J., Amer. J. Clin. Path., 34, (1960),
           313-316.

STEIN'S METHOD TO DEMONSTRATE BILE PIGMENTS

Fixation.   10% formalin.   Fixation should not be pro-
            longed.

SOLUTIONS

1.   Tincture of iodine.

     Iodine crystals   75 gm
     Potassium iodide   50 gm

     Distilled water   50 ml
     95% alcohol to bring volume to   1000 ml

2.   Lugol's iodine (Langeron's double).

     Iodine crystals   1 gm
     Potassium iodide   2 gm
     Distilled water   100 ml

     Dissolve the potassium iodide in a small amount of
     water, then add the iodine crystals. When dissolved,
     add the balance of the water.

3.   Working solution.

     Tincture of iodine   10 ml
     Lugol's iodine   30 ml

4.   Sodium thiosulfate (hypo)   5 gm
     Distilled water   100 ml

5.   Nuclear fast red (Kernechtrot) counterstain. Dis-
     solve 0.1 gm of nuclear fast red in 100 ml of 5%

aqueous aluminum sulfate with the aid of heat. Cool
and filter, add a crystal of thymol.

6. Acetone-xylene 50/50.

PROCEDURE

1. Deparaffinize and hydrate sections to distilled
    water.
2. Stain in working iodine solution for 6 to 12 hours.
3. Wash in distilled water.
4. Decolorize in hypo solution for 15 to 30 seconds.
5. Rinse in distilled water.
6. Counterstain in nuclear fast red for 5 minutes.
7. Rinse in distilled water.
8. Dehydrate quickly in acetone.
9. Clear in acetone-xylene equal parts for 2 minutes.
10. Clear in xylene, two changes.
11. Mount in Permount.

Results.   Bile pigment: green. Nuclei: red.

Ref.   Stein, J.: C. R. Biol., 120 (1935), 1136-1138.

LILLIE'S FERROUS IRON UPTAKE TO DEMONSTRATE MELANIN

Fixation.   10% formalin, absolute alcohol, all chromate
            fixatives should be avoided.

SOLUTIONS

1. Ferrous sulfate solution.

    Ferrous sulfate (FeSo4 7H20)   2.5 gm
    Distilled water   100 ml

2. Potassium ferricyanide solution.

    Potassium ferricyanide (K3Fe(CN)6)   1 gm
    Distilled water   99 ml
    Glacial acetic acid   1 ml

3. Van Gieson's picro-fuchsin.

    Solution A   Solution B
    Acid fuchsin   1 gm   Saturated aqueous solution
    Saturated aqueous   of picric acid (1 to 1.5%)
    solution of picric
    acid   100 ml

To use, combine 1 ml of solution A with 10 ml of solution B.

PROCEDURE

1. Deparaffinize and hydrate sections.
2. Immerse in ferrous sulfate solution for 1 hour.
3. Wash in four to five changes of distilled water for 20 minutes.
4. Place in potassium ferricyanide solution for 30 minutes. (Discard.)
5. Wash in 1% aqueous acetic acid.
6. Counterstain in Van Gieson picro-fuchsin for 1 minute. (Do not use hematoxylin.)
7. Dehydrate in absolute alcohol, two changes, 1 to 2 minutes each.
8. Clear in xylene, two changes.
9. Mount in Permount.

Results. Melanin: dark green. Background: faint green or unstained. With counterstain, collagen usually red; muscle and cytoplasm yellow and brown. Hemosiderin is the only other pigment which reacts with this method, and can be controlled with an iron stain.

Note. Potassium ferrocyanide is unsuitable.

Ref. Lillie, R. D., A. M. A. Arch. Path., 64 (1957), 100-103. Copyright American Medical Association.

LILLIE'S PERFORMIC AND PERACETIC ACID SCHIFF REACTION

Fixation. Fix and section in accordance with the solubility requirements of the lipoid under study. For ceroids, any fixative and paraffin or frozen sections are acceptable. For lipofuchsin pigments, routine formalin and paraffin sections are recommended. For retina and myelin, use formalin or Helly's fluid and paraffin sections.

SOLUTIONS

1. Peracetic acid (add in order given).

   Glacial acetic acid   95.6 ml
   Hydrogen peroxide (30%)   259 ml

Concentrated sulfuric acid   2.2 ml
Allow to stand for 1 to 3 days

Add 40 mg disodium phosphate as stabilizer. Keeps
well at 0.5°C for months.

2.   Performic acid (add in order given).

Formic acid (90%)   8 ml
Hydrogen peroxide (30%)   31 ml
Concentrated sulfuric acid   0.22 ml

Keep at or below 25°C. About 4.7% performic acid is
formed within 2 hours; the solution deteriorates
after a few more hours. Prepare fresh daily.

3.   Normal hydrochloric acid.

Hydrochloric acid, sp. gr. 1.19   83.5 ml
Distilled water   916.5 ml

4.   Schiff reagent. Bring 200 ml of distilled water to
a boil, remove from flame, add 1 gm of basic fuchsin
and stir until dissolved. Cool to 50°C. Filter and
add 20 ml of Normal hydrochloric acid. Cool further
to 25°C. Add 1 gm of sodium or potassium metabisulfite ($Na_2S_2O_5$, $K_2S_2O_5$). Place in the dark in a stoppered bottle for 18 to 24 hours; solution takes on
an orange color. Add 0.5 gm of activated charcoal
and shake well, then filter through a coarse filter
paper. Store under refrigeration in a brown stoppered bottle of the same volume. Solution is stable
for several weeks. Use at room temperature.

5.   Sulfurous acid rinse.

10% sodium metabisulfite   6 ml
Normal hydrochloric acid   5 ml
Distilled water   100 ml

6.   Weigert's iron hematoxylin.

Solution A   Solution B
Iron chloride, 29%   Hematoxylin   1 gm
aqueous   4 ml   95% ethyl
Distilled water   95 ml   alcohol   100 ml
Concentrated hydro-
chloric acid   1 ml

Mix equal parts of A and B immediately prior to use. Solution good only for 24 hours.

7. Saturated aqueous picric acid (approx. 2 gm per 100 ml).

8. Kaiser's glycerin jelly.

Finest gelatin	40 gm
Distilled water	210 ml
Glycerin	250 ml
Carbolic acid crystals	5 gm

Soak the gelatin in the water for 2 hours, add glycerin and carbolic acid. Heat gently for 10 to 15 minutes, stirring constantly until the mixture is smooth; do not allow to burn. (Humason points out that gelatin, when heated above 75°C, may be transformed into metagelatin, and will not harden at room temperature.) Keep in refrigerator and melt in 60°C oven or on water bath before use.

PROCEDURE

1. Deparaffinize and hydrate sections.
2. Remove mercury crystals if necessary.
3. Treat sections with performic acid for 90 minutes or peracetic acid for 2 hours. (This reaction is controlled by omission of the hydrogen peroxide from the performic and peracetic solutions, substituting the same amount of distilled water.)
4. Wash in tap water for 10 minutes.
5. Rinse in distilled water.
6. Place in Schiff solution for 10 minutes. (Discard.)
7. Rinse in three changes of bisulfite rinse for 2 minutes each. (Discard.)
8. Wash in running tap water for 10 minutes.
9. Sections may be counterstained in Weigert's hematoxylin for 1 to 2 minutes. Wash in running tap water 4 to 5 minutes, then counterstain in picric acid for 1 minute.
10. Dehydrate in 95% alcohol, then in absolute alcohol, two changes, 1 to 2 minutes each.
11. Clear in xylene, two changes.
12. Mount in Permount. (If lipids are to be preserved, mount from water into Kaiser's glycerin jelly.)

Results. Ceroid, lipofuchsin pigments, retinal rod acromere, and hair cortex: purple red to magenta. Nuclei: black.

Ref.   Lillie, R. D., Histopathologic Technic and
            Practical Histochemistry, used with permission
            of McGraw-Hill, New York, 1965, 3rd ed.

LILLIE'S METHOD FOR THE DIFFERENTIATION OF MELANIN
AND LIPOFUCHSINS

Fixation. 10% formalin.

SOLUTIONS

1.   Nile blue solution.

     Nile blue A   0.1 gm
     1% aqueous sulfuric acid   100 ml

2.   Kaiser's glycerin jelly.

     Finest gelatin   40 gm
     Distilled water   210 ml
     Glycerin   250 ml
     Carbolic acid crystals   5 gm

     Soak the gelatin in the water for 2 hours, add glyc-
     erin and carbolic acid crystals, and heat gently for
     10 to 15 minutes, stirring constantly until the mix-
     ture is smooth. Keep in refrigerator and melt in
     60°C oven or water bath when needed.

PROCEDURE

1.   Deparaffinize and hydrate sections.
2.   Rinse in distilled water.
3.   Stain in nile blue solution for 30 minutes.
4.   Wash in running tap water for 10 to 20 minutes.
5.   Mount in glycerin jelly.

Results.   Lipofuchsins: dark blue to greenish blue.
            Melanins: dark green. Cytoplasm, muscle: pale
            green. Erythrocytes: greenish yellow to green-
            ish blue. Nuclei: unstained or only faintly
            stained.

Ref.   Lillie, R. D., Stain Tech., 31 (1956A), 151-
            153. Copyright The Williams and Wilkins Co.

FERRIC FERRICYANIDE REDUCTION TECHNIQUE (LILLIE MODIFICATION)

Fixation.   10% formalin. The argentaffin reaction is lost
              with alcoholic fixatives.

SOLUTIONS

1.   Ferric chloride   1 gm
      Distilled water   100 ml

2.   Potassium ferricyanide (K3Fe(CN)6)   1 gm
      Distilled water   100 ml

3.   Working solution.

      Ferric chloride   30 ml
      Potassium ferricyanide   4 ml
      Distilled water   6 ml

      Make up fresh and use within 30 minutes.

4.   1% aqueous acetic acid.

5.   Neutral red counterstain.

      Neutral red   1 gm
      Distilled water   100 ml

PROCEDURE

1.   Deparaffinize and hydrate sections to distilled
      water.
2.   Place sections in working solution for 10 minutes at
      20 to 30°C.
3.   Wash in 1% aqueous acetic acid.
4.   Counterstain in neutral red for 3 minutes.
5.   Dehydrate rapidly through 95% alcohol, then in abso-
      lute alcohol, two changes.
6.   Clear in xylene, two changes.
7.   Mount in Permount.

Results.   Lipofuchsin, melanin, argentaffin granules and
              substances that reduce ferricyanide to ferro-
              cyanide are colored a dark blue. Nuclei: red.

Ref.   Lillie, R. D., Histopathological Technic and
              Practical Histochemistry, used with permission
              of McGraw-Hill, 3rd ed., New York, 1965.

ZIEHL-NEELSEN METHOD FOR ACID-FAST LIPOFUCHSINS

Fixation.   10% formalin for 1 week, a short fixation in
             formalin reduces basophilia.

SOLUTIONS

1.   Carbol fuchsin solution.

      Solution A   Solution B
      Basic fuchsin   0.3 gm   Phenol   5 gm
      95% alcohol   10 ml   Distilled water   95 ml

      When completely dissolved, mix together and filter.

2.   Acid alcohol.

      Hydrochloric acid   1 ml
      70% alcohol   99 ml

3.   Toluidine blue counterstain.

      Toluidine blue   0.5 gm
      Distilled water   100 ml

PROCEDURE

    1.   Deparaffinize and hydrate sections.
    2.   Stain in carbol-fuchsin solution for 3 hours at 60°C.
    3.   Wash in running tap water.
    4.   Differentiate in acid alcohol until red blood cells
          are faintly pink. (Discard.)
    5.   Rinse in water.
    6.   Counterstain in toluidine blue for 30 seconds to 1
          minute.
    7.   Rinse in water.
    8.   Dehydrate in 95% alcohol then absolute alcohol, two
          changes, 1 to 2 minutes each.
    9.   Clear in xylene, two changes.
   10.   Mount in Permount.

Results.   Acid-fast lipofuchsins: bright red. Lipopro-
            teins: pink. Nuclei: blue.

Note.   If counterstaining is too strong the baso-
            philia of the lipofuchsins will lead to devel-
            opment of a purple color in positive lipo-
            fuchsins.

MALLORY'S FUCHSIN METHOD TO DEMONSTRATE HEMOFUCHSIN

<u>Fixation</u>.   10% formalin, alcohol or Helly's fluid.

SOLUTIONS

1.   Mayer's hemalum.

Hematoxylin crystals	1 gm
Sodium iodate	0.2 gm
Aluminum and ammonium sulfate (ammonia alum)	50 gm
Distilled water	1000 ml
Chloral hydrate	50 gm
Citric acid	1 gm

Dissolve hematoxylin, sodium iodate, and ammonia alum overnight in 1000 ml of distilled water. Add chloral hydrate and citric acid. Boil for 5 minutes; when cool, it is ready for use. The solution keeps well.

2.   Basic fuchsin solution.

Basic fuchsin	0.5 gm
Distilled water	50 ml
95% alcohol	50 ml

PROCEDURE

1.   Deparaffinize and hydrate sections.
2.   Remove mercury crystals if necessary.
3.   Stain in Mayer's hemalum solution for 5 minutes.
4.   Wash well in running tap water until blue.
5.   Stain in basic fuchsin solution for 5 to 10 minutes.
6.   Wash in water.
7.   Differentiate in 95% alcohol until no more clouds of stain come off and section is pale pink.
8.   Complete dehydration in absolute alcohol, two changes, 1 to 2 minutes each.
9.   Clear in xylene, two changes.
10. Mount in Permount.

<u>Results</u>.   Nuclei: blue. Hemofuchsin: bright red. Melanin and hemosiderin: unstained in their natural brown colors.

<u>Note</u>.   This method can succeed the Prussian blue method.

Ref.   Mallory, F. B., Pathological Technique, Hafner
              Publishing Co., New York, 1968.

ELFTMAN'S METHOD TO DEMONSTRATE PHOSPHOLIPIDS

Fixation.

              Mercuric chloride 5% aqueous   100 ml
              Potassium dichromate   2.5 gm

              Mix fresh. Fix tissues for 3 days.

SOLUTIONS

1. 0.7 gm of Sudan Black B is dissolved in 100 ml of
    pure propylene glycol by heating to 100° to 110° C
    and is thoroughly stirred for a few minutes. Care
    should be taken not to exceed 110°C, since a useless
    gelatinous mass will result. Filtering the hot solu-
    tion through a Whatman No. 2 paper removes most of
    theundissolved impurities. After cooling to room tem-
    perature it is filtered again through a fritted glass
    filter of medium porosity with the aid of suction.

2. 85% propylene glycol.

    Pure propylene glycol   85 ml
    Distilled water   15 ml

3. Kaiser's glycerin jelly.

    Finest gelatin   40 gm
    Distilled water   210 ml
    Glycerin   250 ml
    Carbolic acid crystals   5 gm

    Soak the gelatin in water for 2 hours, add glycerin
    and carbolic acid. Heat gently for 10 to 15 minutes,
    stirring constantly until the mixture is smooth; do
    not allow to burn. (Humason points out that gelatin,
    when heated above 75°C may be transformed into meta-
    gelatin, which will not harden at room temperature.)
    Keep in refrigerator and melt in 60°C oven or on
    water bath before use.

PROCEDURE

1. Deparaffinize and hydrate sections through to absolute alcohol.
2. Place in pure propylene glycol for 5 minutes.
3. Stain in Sudan black solution for 30 minutes.
4. Differentiate in 85% propylene glycol for 2 to 3 minutes. (Discard.)
5. Wash in distilled water.
6. Mount in Kaiser's glycerin jelly.

Results.   Phospholipids: black.

Ref.   Elftman, H., Stain Tech., 32 (1957B), 29-31.
            Copyright The Williams and Wilkins Co.

SCHULTZ'S MODIFICATION OF LIEBERMANN-BURCHARDT METHOD TO DEMONSTRATE CHOLESTEROL

Fixation.   10% formalin.

SOLUTIONS

1. Iron alum solution.

Iron alum (ferric ammonium sulfate)	2.5 gm
Distilled water	100 ml

2. Acetic-sulfuric acid mixture. Prepare just before use.

Glacial acetic acid	2-5 ml
Sulfuric acid	2-5 ml

    Mix the sulfuric acid with the acetic acid in a test tube in an ice bath. This reaction may be violet at room temperature.

PROCEDURE

1. Cut frozen sections and place them in the iron alum solution for 3 days at 37°C.
2. Rinse in distilled water.
3. Mount sections on slides and blot dry with fine filter paper.
4. Cover section with a few drops of acetic-sulfuric acid mixture.
5. Cover slip and remove excess fluid; examine immediately or within 5 minutes. Cover glass may be

sealed with petrolatum. Section is good for 30
minutes.

Results.   The blue-green color that forms within a few
            minutes is characteristic of cholesterol and
            its esters. Adrenal cortex may be used as a
            control.

Ref.   McManus, J. F. A. and Mowry, R. W., Staining
            Methods Histologic and Histochemical, Harper &
            Row, New York, 1960.

PUTT'S FLAMING RED METHOD TO DEMONSTRATE LIPIDS

Fixation.   10% formalin.

SOLUTIONS

1.   Pure propylene glycol.

2.   Flaming red solution. Dissolve 1 gm of flaming red*
      in 100 ml of pure propylene glycol. Heat the solu-
      tion gently, stirring constantly, to 95 to 100°C.
      No not exceed 100°C, since a useless gelatinous mass
      will result. Filter the solution, while still hot,
      through a Whatman No. 2 filter paper. This removes
      most of the excess dye and undissolved impurities.
      After cooling overnight at room temperature, filter
      again through a fritted glass filter of medium po-
      rosity with the aid of suction. If the solution be-
      comes turbid on standing, it should be refiltered.
      The glycol solvents should be obtained in as nearly
      pure a form as possible, since any appreciable water
      content (30 to 40%) will prevent much of the dye
      from going into solution.

3.   Differentiator.

      Pure propylene glycol   85 ml
      Distilled water   15 ml

4.   Bullard's hematoxylin.

      50% alcohol   144 ml
      Glacial acetic acid   16 ml

*Flaming red, C. I. No. 12085, Fisher Scientific Co.
 Burnstone, M. S., Amer. J. Clin. Path., 28 (1957B),
 429-430.

Hematoxylin crystals	8 gm

Heat and add:

Distilled water	250 ml
Aluminum and ammonium sulfate (ammonia alum)	20 gm

Heat to a boil and add slowly:

Mercuric oxide (red)	8 gm

Cool quickly, filter and add:

95% alcohol	275 ml
Glycerin	330 ml
Glacial acetic acid	18 ml
Aluminum and ammonium sulfate	40 gm

Can be used at once and lasts for years.

5.   Kaiser's glycerin jelly.

Finest gelatin	40 gm
Distilled water	210 ml
Glycerin	250 ml
Carbolic acid crystals	5 gm

Soak the gelatin in water for 2 hours, add glycerin and carbolic acid. Heat gently for 10 to 15 minutes, stirring constantly until the mixture is smooth; do not allow to burn. (Humason points out that gelatin, when heated above 75°C, may be transformed into meta-gelatin, which will not harden at room temperature.) Keep in refrigerator and melt in 60°C oven or on water bath before use.

PROCEDURE

1.   Cut frozen sections at 10 to 15 microns and collect in distilled water.
2.   With a glass "hockey stick" place the sections in fresh distilled water for 2 to 3 minutes.
3.   Place in pure propylene glycol and agitate gently for 2 to 3 minutes.
4.   Transfer to flaming red solution for 5 to 6 minutes; agitate gently.
5.   Differentiate in 85% glycol solution for 1 to 2 minutes. (Discard.)
6.   Wash in distilled water for 1 minute.
7.   Stain nuclei in Bullard's hematoxylin for 1 minute.

8. Rinse in tap water.
9. Rinse in weak ammonia water until no more blue clouds
    of stain come off. (Tap water 50 ml   28% ammonium
    hydroxide 3 to 4 drops.)
10. Wash in tap water. (Sections may be left at this
    point until ready for mounting.)
11. Mount in Kaiser's glycerin jelly.

Results.   Lipids and mitochondria: varying shades of red.
             Nuclei: blue.

Note.   Acid alcohol differentiation is omitted as
             some lipids may be removed.

             Petri and Stender dishes are convenient glass-
             ware in which to carry out this type of stain-
             ing.

             *Burnstone's solution is recommended as a sub-
             stitute for Kaiser's glycerin jelly and may be
             used at room temperature.

             50 gm of polyvinyl pyrrolidone (PVP) Plasdone
             C† are dissolved in 50 ml of distilled water
             and permitted to stand overnight. 2 ml of
             glycerin are then added and the mixture stirred.
             A crystal of thymol may be added as a preserva-
             tive.

Ref.   Putt, F. A., Lab. Invest., 5 (1956), 377-379.
             Copyright The Williams & Wilkins Co.

CHIFFELLE AND PUTT PROPYLENE GLYCOL METHOD TO
DEMONSTRATE LIPIDS

Fixation. 10% formalin.

SOLUTIONS

1. Pure propylene glycol.

2. Propylene glycol dye solution. Seven tenths of a
    gram of Sudan IV, oil red O or Sudan Black B is dis-
    solved in 100 ml of pure propylene glycol by heating
    to 95 to 100°C and thoroughly stirring for a few

*Burnstone, M. S. , Amer. J. Clin. Path., 28 (1957B), 429-
430.
†Plasdone C, General Dyestuffs Corporation.

minutes. Care should be taken not to exceed 100°C,
since a useless gelatinous mass will result. Filter-
ing the hot solution through a Whatman No. 2 paper
removes most of the excess dye and undissolved impurities. After cooling to room temperature, filter
it again through a fritted glass filter of medium po-
rosity with the aid of suction. As an alternative
the solution may be filtered through paper for a
second time, but the procedure is long because of
the viscosity of the glycols. The glycol solvents
should be obtained in as nearly a pure form as possible, since an appreciable water content (30 to 40%)
will prevent much of the dye from going into solution.

3.   Pure propylene glycol   85 ml
      Distilled water   15 ml

4.   Bullard's hematoxylin.

      50% alcohol   144 ml
      Glacial acetic acid   16 ml
      Hematoxylin crystals   8 gm

      Heat and add:

      Distilled water   250 ml
      Aluminum and ammonium sulfate
      (ammonium alum)   20 gm

      Heat to a boil and add slowly:

      Mercuric oxide (red)   8 gm

      Cool quickly, filter and add:

      95% alcohol   275 ml
      Glycerin   330 ml
      Glacial acetic acid   18 ml
      Aluminum and ammonium sulfate   40 gm

5.   Kaiser's glycerin jelly.

      Finest gelatin   40 gm
      Distilled water   210 ml
      Glycerin   250 ml
      Carbolic acid crystals   5 gm

      Soak the gelatin in water for 2 hours, add glycerin
      and carbolic acid. Heat gently for 10 to 15 minutes,
      stirring constantly until the mixture is smooth; do

not allow to burn. (Humason* points out that gelatin, when heated about 75°C, may be transformed into
metagelatin, which will not harden at room temperature.) Keep in refrigerator and melt in 60°C oven
or on water bath before use.

PROCEDURE

1. Cut frozen sections at 10 to 15 microns into distilled water.
2. Transfer to fresh distilled water with a glass
   "hockey stick."
3. Dehydrate sections in pure propylene glycol for 3 to
   5 minutes; agitate sections gently.
4. Rinse in distilled water.
5. Sudan Black B stained sections are not counterstained, but are mounted directly in glycerin jelly.
6. Sudan IV or oil red O sections are counterstained in
   Bullard's hematoxylin.
7. Rinse in distilled water.
8. Rinse in weak ammonia water until no more clouds of
   color come off. (Tap water 50 ml; Ammonium hydroxide 28% 3 to 4 drops.)
9. Rinse in tap water. (Sections may be left here until
   ready for mounting.)
10. Mount in Kaiser's glycerin jelly.

Results.   Sudan Black B stained sections: fat black on a
            blue-gray background. Sudan or oil red O sec-
            tions: fat red; nuclei blue. This method
            demonstrates total lipid content of cells.

Ref.   Chiffelle, T. L. and Putt, F. A., Stain Tech.
            26 (1951), 51-56. Copyright the Williams and
            Wilkins Co.

LILLIE AND ASHBURN'S SUPERSATURATED ISOPROPANOL
METHOD FOR LIPID

Fixation. 10% formalin.

SOLUTIONS

1. Stock solution.

   99% Isopropanol   100 ml
   Oil red-O   250-500 mg

*Humason, G. L., Animal Tissue Techniques, W. H. Freeman
& Co., San Francisco, 1962.

2.   Working solution.

      Dilute 6 ml of stock solution with 4 ml of water.
      Let stand for 10 to 15 minutes and filter. Usable
      for several hours.

3.   Mayer's hemalum.

Hematoxylin crystals	1 gm
Sodium iodate	0.2 gm
Aluminum and ammonium sulfate (ammonia alum)	50 gm
Distilled water	1000 ml
Chloral hydrate	50 gm
Citric acid	1 gm

      Dissolve hematoxylin, sodium iodate, and ammonium
      alum overnight in 1000 ml of distilled water; add
      chloral hydrate and citric acid. Boil for 5 min-
      utes; when cool, it is ready for use. The solution
      keeps well.

4. | | |
      |---|---:|
      | Disodium phosphate | 1 gm |
      | Distilled water | 100 ml |

5.   Kaiser's glycerin jelly. Soak the gelatin in water
      for 2 hours, add glycerin and carbolic acid. Heat
      gently for 10 to 15 minutes, stirring constantly
      until the mixture is smooth; do not allow to burn.
      (Humason points out that gelatin, when heated above
      75°C, may be transformed into metagelatin, which
      will not harden at room temperature.) Keep in re-
      frigerator and melt in 60°C oven or on water bath
      before use.

PROCEDURE

1.   Cut frozen sections at 10 microns into distilled
      water.
2.   With a glass "hockey stick" transfer to working solu-
      tion for 10 minutes.
3.   Rinse in water.
4.   Stain nuclei in Mayer's hemalum.
5.   Blue nuclei in disodium phosphate.
6.   Wash in water and mount on slide in Kaiser's glycerin
      jelly.

Results.   Fats and lipofuchsins: brilliant red.   Nuclei:
           blue.

Ref.   Lillie, R. D., Histopathologic Technic and
           Practical Histochemistry, 3rd ed., used with
           permission of McGraw-Hill, New York, 1943.

HERXHEIMER'S METHOD TO DEMONSTRATE LIPID

Fixation. 10% formalin.

SOLUTIONS

1.   70% alcohol.

2.   Herxheimer's staining solution.

     Sudan IV, flaming red or oil red O   1 gm
     70% alcohol   50 ml
     Acetone   50 ml

     Shake well; allow excess dye to settle overnight in
     a stoppered bottle. Do not filter. The solution
     should be stored in a well-stoppered bottle to pre-
     vent evaporation. This is a saturated solution; do
     not agitate before use, as suspended dye particles
     will cause precipitate to form on sections.

3.   Bullard's hematoxylin.

     50% alcohol   144 ml
     Glacial acetic acid   16 ml
     Hematoxylin crystals   8 gm

     Heat and add:

     Distilled water   250 ml
     Aluminum and ammonium sulfate
     (ammonium alum)   20 gm

     Heat to a boil and add slowly:

     Mercuric oxide (red)   8 gm

     Cool quickly, filter, and add:

     95% alcohol   275 ml
     Glycerin   330 ml
     Glacial acetic acid   18 ml

Aluminum and ammonium sulfate   40 gm

4.   Kaiser's glycerin jelly.*

Finest gelatin   40 gm
Distilled water   210 ml
Glycerin   250 ml
Carbolic acid crystals   5 gm

Soak the gelatin in water for 2 hours, add glycerin
and carbolic acid. Heat gently for 10 to 15 minutes, stirring constantly until the mixture is
smooth; do not allow to burn. (Humason points out
that gelatin, when heated above 75°C, may be transformed into metagelatin, which will not harden at
room temperature.) Keep in refrigerator and melt
in 60°C oven or on water bath before use.

PROCEDURE

 1. Cut frozen sections at 10 to 15 microns and collect
     in distilled water.
 2. With a glass "hockey stick" transfer sections to
     fresh distilled water and wash for 3 to 5 minutes.
 3. Rinse the sections briefly in 70% alcohol; keep the
     dish covered.
 4. Transfer sections to Herxheimer's solution for 5
     minutes. The staining should be carried out in a
     covered Stender dish to prevent evaporation of ace-
     tone. Otherwise, dye crystals will form in the fin-
     ished section in 2 to 3 days. A number of sections
     may be stained in the same solution, which is dis-
     carded.
 5. Rinse quickly in 70% alcohol to remove excess stain.
 6. Counterstain in Bullard's hematoxylin for 1 to 2
     minutes.
 7. Rinse in distilled water.
 8. Rinse in weak ammonia water until no more clouds
     come off. (Tap water 50 ml. Ammonium hydroxide 28%
     3 to 4 drops.)
 9. Rinse well in tap water.
10. Mount in Kaiser's glycerin jelly.

Results.   Lipid: red. Nuclei: blue. Fatty acids un-
            stained.

*Prepared glycerin jelly, Hartmann-Leddon Co., Philadel-
phia, Pa.

Note.   Many histological laboratories still employ
             this procedure in spite of the fact that many
             lipids are removed by the acetone-alcohol dye
             solvent.

Ref.   Mallory, F. B. Pathological Technique Hafner
             Publishing Co; New York, 1968.

CAIN'S NILE BLUE SULFATE TO DEMONSTRATE NEUTRAL FATS

Fixation. 10% formalin.

SOLUTIONS

1.   Nile blue A   1.5 gm
      Distilled water   100 ml

2.   1% aqueous glacial acetic acid.

3.   Kaiser's glycerin jelly.

      Finest gelatin   40 gm
      Distilled water   210 ml
      Glycerin   250 ml
      Carbolic acid crystals   5 gm

      Soak the gelatin in water for 2 hours, add glycerin
      and carbolic acid. Heat gently for 10 to 15 min-
      utes, stirring constantly until the mixture is
      smooth; do not allow to burn. (Humason points out
      that gelatin, when heated above 75°C, may be trans-
      formed into metagelatin, which will not harden at
      room temperature.) Keep in refrigerator and melt in
      60°C oven or on water bath before use.

PROCEDURE

1.   Cut frozen sections at 10 to 15 microns into dis-
      tilled water.
2.   Rinse in fresh distilled water.
3.   Stain in Nile blue solution for 20 minutes.
4.   Rinse in tap water.
5.   Differentiate in 1% acetic acid for 1 to 20 minutes
      until pink is clear.
6.   Wash well in several changes of distilled water.

7.   Mount in Kaiser's glycerin jelly.

Results.   Neutral fats: pink to red. Fatty acids: blue
            to violet. Nuclei and elastic tissue: dark
            blue.

Note.   This method is not considered specific for
         fatty acids; acidic lipids with a high melting
         point may be demonstrated by raising the tem-
         perature of the solutions in steps 3, 4, and 5
         to 70°C.

Ref.   Lillie, R. D., Histopathologic Technic and
        Practical Histochemistry, 3rd ed., used
        with permission of McGraw-Hill, New York,
        1965.

FELTON'S METHOD FOR THE IDENTIFICATION OF
LIPIDOL IN TISSUE SECTIONS

Fixation. 10% formalin.

SOLUTIONS

1.   Brilliant cresyl blue solution.

      Brilliant cresyl blue   0.5 gm
      Normal saline   100 ml

2.   Silver nitrate solution.

      Silver nitrate   10 gm
      Distilled water   100 ml

3.   Kaiser's glycerin jelly.

      Finest gelatin   40 gm
      Distilled water   210 ml
      Glycerin   250 ml
      Carbolic acid crystals   5 gm

      Soak the gelatin in water for 2 hours, add glycerin
      and carbolic acid. Heat gently for 10 to 15 min-
      utes, stirring constantly until the mixture is
      smooth; do not allow to burn. (Humason points out

that gelatin, when heated above 75°C, may be transformed into metagelatin, which will not harden at
room temperature.) Keep in refrigerator and melt in
60°C oven or on water bath before use.

PROCEDURE

 1. Wash tissue blocks in running water for 30 minutes.
 2. Embed in 10% gelatin and cool in refrigerator.
 3. Cut and trim gelatin blocks and place in 10% forma-
     lin for 24 hours.
 4. Wash gelatin block for 20 minutes in tap water.
 5. Cut frozen sections at 15 microns into distilled
     water; rinse well.
 6. Transfer sections to brilliant cresyl blue solution
     for 2 minutes.
 7. Wash well in distilled water.
 8. Transfer sections to silver nitrate solution for 2
     minutes.
 9. Wash well in distilled water.
10. Mount sections on slide and drain.
11. Mount in Kaiser's glycerin jelly.

Results.   Lipidol behaves as a halogenated hydrocarbon
            in that it forms a yellow precipitate, silver
            iodide on treatment with silver nitrate in aque-
            ous solutions in the cold. In frozen sections
            containing lipidol treated with silver nitrate
            the oil droplets assume a yellow-brown appear-
            ance. In such sections, stained first with
            brilliant cresyl blue and then treated with sil-
            ver nitrate, the lipidol droplets assume a
            dark brown fairly homogenous aspect. In sec-
            tions of subcutaneous fat and "golden pneumonia"
            stained with brilliant cresyl blue and then
            treated with silver nitrate the fat particles
            are unchanged, maintaining their pink to violet
            color.

Ref.   Felton, W. L., Lab. Invest., 1 (1952), 364-367.
            Copyright The Williams and Wilkins Co.

SCHULTZ'S METHOD TO DEMONSTRATE SODIUM URATE

Fixation. Absolute alcohol. Tissue section should be thin.

SOLUTIONS

1. Carmine solution.

Distilled water	128 ml
Lithium carbonate	1 gm
Carmine	2 gm
Ammonium chloride	4 gm

    Boil for a few minutes. Cool, make up to original
    volume with distilled water, and add:

Ammonium hydroxide 28%	12 ml

2. Working solution (discard after use):

Carmine solution	30 ml
Methyl alcohol	25 ml
Ammonium hydroxide 28%	4 ml
Distilled water	11 ml

3. Methylene blue solution.

Methylene blue	1 gm
Absolute alcohol	100 ml

4. Picric acid, saturated aqueous
    solution (about 1 to 1 1/2%)   27 ml
    Sodium sulfate, saturated aqueous
    solution (about 50%)   3 ml

PROCEDURE

1. Dehydrate tissue blocks in three changes of acetone,
    2 hours each.
2. Place in acetone-benzene 50/50 for 30 minutes.
3. Clear in two changes of benzene, 30 minutes each.
4. Infiltrate with paraffin in vacuum oven, two changes,
    30 minutes each.
5. Embed and cut paraffin sections as usual.
6. Deparaffinize sections to absolute alcohol.
7. Stain in carmine working solution for 5 minutes;
    keep slide in motion continuously during staining.
8. Rinse in several changes of absolute alcohol.
9. Stain in methylene blue solution for 30 seconds.
10. Rinse in several changes of absolute alcohol.
11. Stain in picric acid-sodium sulfate solution for 30
    seconds, keeping slides in motion.
12. Dehydrate in several changes of absolute alcohol.
13. Clear in xylene, two changes.
14. Mount in Permount.

Results.   Nuclei are stained a grayish blue. Cytoplasm:
           yellowish. Uric acid: deep blue green. Mono-
           sodium urate: brilliant green.

Ref.   Lillie, R. D., Histopathologic Technic and
           Practical Histochemistry, 3rd ed., used with
           permission of McGraw-Hill, New York, 1965,
           p. 256.

MALLORY'S ALUM HEMATOXYLIN METHOD TO DEMONSTRATE
SODIUM URATE

Fixation. Absolute alcohol.

SOLUTIONS

1.   Mayer's hemalum (modified).

        Hematoxylin   1 gm
        Distilled water   1000 ml
        Sodium iodate   0.2 gm
        Aluminum and ammonium sulfate
        (ammonia alum)   50 gm
        Chloral hydrate   50 gm

     Dissolve the hematoxylin in water with the aid of
     gentle heat. Add the sodium iodate, then the alum;
     stir until the alum is dissolved and then add the
     chloral hydrate. Do not add citric acid as usual.

PROCEDURE

1.   Deparaffinize and hydrate sections.
2.   Place sections for 1 to 2 minutes in cold hematoxy-
     lin solution.
3.   Rinse quickly in cold water.
4.   Dehydrate in 95% alcohol, 1 minute.
5.   Dehydrate in absolute alcohol, two changes, 1 to 2
     minutes each.
6.   Clear in xylene, two changes.
7.   Mount in Permount.

Results.   Sodium urate crystals and nuclei: deep blue.

Ref.   Mallory, F. B., Pathological Technique, Hafner
           Publishing Co., New York, 1968.

SODIUM RHODIZONATE METHOD TO DEMONSTRATE BARIUM SALTS

<u>Fixation</u>. 10% formalin.

SOLUTIONS

1.   Sodium rhodizonate* (prepare
      fresh each time)   0.2 gm
      Distilled water   100 ml

2.   Hydrochloric acid   20 ml
      Distilled water   80 ml

PROCEDURE

1.   Deparaffinize and hydrate sections to distilled water.
2.   Place in a freshly prepared solution of sodium rho-
      dizonate in 60°C oven for 1 to 2 hours, in covered
      Coplin jar.
3.   Rinse quickly in distilled water.
4.   If desired, convert the black rhodizonate to red
      salt by placing in hydrochloric acid solution for
      2 to 3 minutes.
5.   Wash in water.
6.   Dehydrate in 95% alcohol, then in absolute alcohol,
      two changes, 1 to 2 minutes each.
7.   Clear in xylene, two changes.
8.   Mount in Permount.

<u>Results</u>.   Barium deposits: black, or converted to red by
            acid treatment. Strontium salts, which react
            similarly, would be dissolved by this treatment.

<u>Ref</u>.   Pearce, A. G. E., Histochemistry, Theoretical
            and Applied, 2nd ed., Little, Brown and Co.,
            Boston, 1960.

VON KOSSA'S METHOD TO DEMONSTRATE CALCIUM

<u>Fixation</u>. 10% buffered formalin or absolute alcohol.
           (Avoid calcium-containing fixatives.)

SOLUTIONS

1.   Silver nitrate solution.

      Silver nitrate (prepare fresh)   5 gm
      Distilled water   100 ml

*Sodium rhodizonate, Fisher Scientific Co.

2.   Sodium thiosulfate   5 gm
     Distilled water   100 ml

3.   Nuclear fast red (Kernechtrot) counterstain.

     Nuclear fast red   0.1 gm
     Aluminum sulfate 5% aqueous   100 ml

     Dissolve with the aid of heat. Cool and filter;
     add a crystal of thymol. Solution keeps well at
     room temperature; filter before use.

PROCEDURE

1.   Deparaffinize and hydrate sections to distilled
     water. (Use control slide.)
2.   Place sections in silver nitrate solution in a cov-
     ered Coplin jar for 10 to 60 minutes and expose to
     light (60-W bulb) or indirect sunlight.
3.   Wash thoroughly in distilled water.
4.   Reduce for a few minutes in sodium thiosulfate to
     remove excess silver nitrate.
5.   Rinse in distilled water.
6.   Counterstain in nuclear fast red for 5 minutes.
7.   Rinse in water.
8.   Dehydrate in 95% alcohol, then absolute alcohol, two
     changes, 1 to 2 minutes each.
9.   Clear in xylene, two changes.
10. Mount in Permount.

Results.   Calcium is stained a deep black where it occurs
           in masses; finely dispersed granules do not
           stain deeply. Nuclei: red.

Note.   All glassware should be chemically clean.

Ref.   Lillie, R. D., Histopathologic Technic and
           Practical Histochemistry, used with permission
           of McGraw-Hill, New York, 1965.

SCHUJENINOFF'S TEST FOR CALCIUM DEPOSITS

Fixation. 10% buffered formalin. (Avoid calcium contain-
           ing fixatives.)

SOLUTIONS

1.   Sulfuric acid   5 ml
     Distilled water   100 ml

PROCEDURE

1.   Deparaffinize and leave in absolute alcohol.
2.   Rinse in acetone.
3.   Allow section to dry at room temperature.
4.   Cover section with a loose cover glass and draw a
      drop of 5% sulfuric acid under the cover glass;
      examine under low power of the microscope.

Results. Calcium is indicated if long thin needles are
          formed. These needles are hydrated calcium
          sulfate and, if present, will gradually change
          to prisms and finally to piles of rectangular
          plates.

Ref.   Schujeninoff, S., Heilk., 18 (1897), 79.

ALIZARIN RED S METHOD TO DEMONSTRATE CALCIUM

Fixation. 10% buffered formalin. (Avoid calcium-contain-
           ing fixatives.)

SOLUTIONS

1.   Alizarin red S solution.

      Alizarin red S   0.1 gm
      Distilled water   100 ml

2.   Light green SF yellowish solution.

      Light green SF yellowish   0.1 gm
      Distilled water   100 ml

3.   Glacial acetic acid   1 ml
      Distilled water   99 ml

PROCEDURE

1.   Deparaffinize sections to distilled water. (Run
      control slide.)
2.   Stain in alizarin solution at room temperature for
      1 hour.
3.   Rinse in distilled water.
4.   Counterstain in light green for 30 seconds.
5.   Rinse quickly in 1% acetic acid solution.
6.   Blot dry with fine filter paper.
7.   Decolorize rapidly in absolute alcohol.
8.   Clear in xylene.
9.   Mount in Permount.

Results.   Nuclei: pale green.   Calcium deposits: bright
           red.

Ref.   Dahl, L. K., Proc. Soc. Exp. Biol. Med., 80
           (1952), 474-479.

GRANDIS' AND MAININI'S PURPURIN METHOD TO
DEMONSTRATE CALCIUM

Fixation. Buffered 10% formalin or absolute alcohol.
           (Avoid calcium-containing fixatives.)

SOLUTIONS

1.   Purpurin solution.*   Purpurin, saturated solution
      in absolute alcohol, about 0.7%.

2.   Sodium chloride solution.

      Sodium chloride   0.75 gm
      Distilled water   100 ml

3.   70% alcohol.

PROCEDURE

1.   Deparaffinize sections to absolute alcohol.   (Run
      control slide.)
2.   Stain in purpurin solution in a Coplin jar for 5
      minutes.
3.   Immerse in sodium chloride solution for 5 minutes.
4.   Wash in 70% alcohol until stain ceases to come off
      sections.
5.   Dehydrate in 95% alcohol.
6.   Dehydrate in absolute alcohol.
7.   Clear in xylene.
8.   Mount in Permount.

Results.   Calcium deposits: red.

Note.   The presence of massive deposits of uric acid
           and its salts, which stain like phosphate-car-
           bonate, can be a source of error, but the latter
           are removed by washing the deparaffinized sec-
           tions for 1 minute in a 1% aqueous solution of
           hydrochloric acid.

*Purpurin, C. I. No. 58205, ESBE Laboratories, Toronto,
 Ontario

Ref.   Grandis, V. and Mainini, C., Arch. Ital. Biol.
            34 (1900), 73-78.

BUNTING'S METHOD TO DEMONSTRATE IRON WITH PRUSSIAN
BLUE REACTION

Fixation. 10% buffered formalin. (Iron deposits in
          Helly or Zenker's fixed material will appear
          diffuse.)

SOLUTIONS

1.   Potassium or sodium ferrocyanide   2 gm
      Distilled water   100 ml

2.   Hydrochloric acid   2 ml
      Distilled water   100 ml

3.   Working solution. Equal parts of the solutions
      above. The solutions of Prussian blue are unstable,
      turning pale green after an hour or so; they should
      always be made immediately before use and filtered.

4.   Nuclear fast red (Kernechtrot) counterstain.

      Nuclear fast red   0.1 gm
      Aluminum sulfate 5% aqueous   100 ml

      Dissolve with the aid of heat. Cool and filter, add
      crystal of thymol. Solution keeps well at room tem-
      perature; filter before use.

PROCEDURE

1.   Deparaffinize and hydrate sections to distilled
      water. (Run control slide.)
2.   Place sections in working solution of hydrochloric
      acid-ferrocyanide for 1 hour at room temperature,
      changing solution at end of first half hour.
3.   Rinse in distilled water.
4.   Counterstain in Nuclear fast red for 5 minutes.
5.   Rinse in distilled water.
6.   Dehydrate in 95% alcohol, then in absolute alcohol,
      two changes, 1 to 2 minutes each.
7.   Clear in xylene, two changes.
8.   Mount in Permount.

Results. Nuclei: red. Ferric iron: blue.

Note.   All glassware used for the stain should be
            chemically clean and rinsed in distilled water.
            If small amounts of iron are to be detected,
            do not counterstain; use a pink filter on the
            light source. Iron stains are not permanent
            and fade after a few weeks; according to Gomori,
            this is due to reduction. The color can be re-
            stored quickly by exposing the sections to air
            or, even better, to dilute hydrogen peroxide.
            The tissue flotation bath should also contain
            distilled water.

Ref.   Bunting, H., Stain Tech., 24 (1949), 109-115.
            Copyright The Williams and Wilkins Co.

TURNBULL BLUE METHOD TO DEMONSTRATE FERROUS IRON

Fixation. 10% buffered formalin. (Iron deposits in
          Helly or Zenker's fixed material will appear
          diffuse.)

SOLUTIONS

1.   Ammonium sulfide solution.

      Ammonium sulfide   10 ml
      Distilled water   90 ml

2.   Potassium ferricyanide.

      Potassium ferricyanide   20 gm
      Distilled water   100 ml

3.   Hydrochloric acid.

      Hydrochloric acid   1 ml
      Distilled water   99 ml

4.   Working solution. Equal parts of potassium ferri-
      cyanide and hydrochloric acid solutions.

5.   Basic fuchsin counterstain.

      Basic fuchsin   0.5 gm
      Absolute alcohol   50 ml
      Distilled water   50 ml

PROCEDURE

  1. Deparaffinize and hydrate sections to distilled

water.   (Run control slide.)
2. Transfer to ammonium sulfide solution for 1 hour at room temperature in a glass Coplin dish with a tightly fitting cover.
3. Wash thoroughly in distilled water.
4. Place in working solution of hydrochloric acid-potassium ferricyanide for 10 to 20 minutes to convert the ferrosulfide which is formed into Turnbull blue. Discard solution.
5. Wash well in distilled water.
6. Counterstain in fuchsin solution for 5 to 10 minutes.
7. Wash in distilled water.
8. Differentiate in 95% alcohol, then in absolute alcohol, two changes, 1 to 2 minutes each.
9. Clear in xylene, two changes.
10. Mount in Permount.

Results.   Nuclei and hemofuchsin granules: bright red. Ferrous irons: blue.

Note.   The tissue flotation bath should contain distilled water.

Ref.   Bunting, H., Stain Tech. 24 (1949), 109-115. Copyright The Williams and Wilkins Co.

MODIFIED MALLORY HEMATOXYLIN METHOD TO DEMONSTRATE HEMOSIDERIN IRON

Fixation. 10% buffered formalin, absolute alcohol.

SOLUTIONS

1.   Ammonium sulfide solution.

     Ammonium sulfide   10 ml
     Distilled water   90 ml

2.   Hematoxylin solution. Dissolve 5 to 10 mg of ether-washed hematoxylin crystals in a few ml of absolute alcohol; to this add about twice the volume of boiled distilled water.

3.   Ether   50 ml
     Absolute alcohol   50 ml

4.   Nuclear fast red (Kernechtrot) counterstain.

     Nuclear fast red   0.1 gm
     Aluminum sulfate 5% aqueous   100 ml

Dissolve with the aid of heat. Cool and filter;
add a crystal of thymol. Solution keeps well at
room temperature. Filter before use.

PROCEDURE

1. Deparaffinize and hydrate sections to distilled
    water. (Run a control slide.)
2. Expose to ammonium sulfide at room temperature for
    1 hour in a well covered Coplin jar.
3. Rinse in distilled water.
4. Stain in hematoxylin solution for 1 to 2 hours.
5. Rinse off excess hematoxylin in ether-alcohol
    mixture.
6. Rinse in distilled water.
7. Counterstain if desired in nuclear fast red for 5
    minutes.
8. Rinse in distilled water.
9. Dehydrate in 95% alcohol, then in absolute alcohol,
    two changes, 1 to 2 minutes each.
10. Clear in xylene, two changes.
11. Mount in Permount.

Results.   Hemosiderin: blue-black. Nuclei: red.

Note.   Hemosiderin iron, whether fixed in formalin or
             in alcohol, may be stained an unsatisfactory
             brown, while interstitial iron is a blue-black
             with hematoxylin. If the section is exposed to
             ammonium sulfide, however, hemosiderin iron is
             stained blue-black or gray. After such pre-
             treatment it is clearly seen that the pale
             brown objects (iron sulfide) are the ones that
             react with hematoxylin. Thus the specificity
             of the procedure in the particular specimen
             can be controlled.

Ref.   Bunting, H., Stain Tech., 24 (1949), 109-115.
             Copyright The Williams and Wilkins Co.

HUKILL AND PUTT'S REACTION TO DEMONSTRATE IRON

Fixation. 10% buffered formalin.

SOLUTIONS

1. Bathophenanthroline solution.* Add 100 mg of bath-
    ophenanthroline to 100 ml of 3% glacial acetic acid.

*Bathophenanthroline, G. Frederick Smith Chemical Co.,
Columbus, Ohio.

Agitate and warm overnight at 50 to 60°C. Cool to room temperature, add 0.5 ml of thioglycolic acid and filter. This solution is stable for 4 weeks, but the thioglycolic acid*should be replenished before each use, as it is rapidly oxidized on exposure to air.

2. Methylene blue counterstain.

Methylene blue   0.5 gm
Distilled water   100 ml

PROCEDURE

1. Embed tissue in paraffin.
2. Cut sections at 5 microns and float on distilled water. (Run a control slide.)
3. Deparaffinize and hydrate sections to distilled water.
4. Stain in bathophenanthroline solution for 2 hours.
5. Rinse in distilled water.
6. Counterstain in methylene blue for 3 minutes.
7. Rinse in three changes of distilled water, 1 minute each.
8. Dry in 60°C oven until thoroughly dehydrated.
9. Mount in Permount.

Results. Iron: red. Nuclei: blue.

Note. Glass-distilled water must be used in all solutions. Glassware should be acid-cleaned and rinsed in distilled water.

Ref. Hukill, P. B. and Putt, F. A., J. Histochem. Cytochem., 10 (1962), 490-494. Copyright The Williams and Wilkins Co.

ELFTMAN METHOD TO DEMONSTRATE GOLD IN TISSUE

Fixation. 10% buffered formalin.

SOLUTIONS

1. 3% hydrogen peroxide.

*Thioglycolic acid, The Matheson Co., East Rutherford, New Jersey.

PROCEDURE

1.   Cut paraffin sections at 10 microns.
2.   Deparaffinize and hydrate sections to distilled
      water.
3.   Place sections in hydrogen peroxide solution in 37°C
      oven for 1 to 3 days.
4.   Wash sections in distilled water.
5.   Dehydrate in 95% alcohol, then in absolute alcohol,
      two changes, 1 to 2 minutes each.
6.   Clear in xylene, two changes.
7.   Mount in Permount.

Results.   Gold in tissue is reduced to the metallic form
           by the peroxide solution, and displays the
           range of colors of colloidal gold: rose and
           purple granules. The peroxide bleaches the
           interfering pigments. Since no metallic ions
           have been added, the confusion arising from in-
           cidental deposits of metals is eliminated.

Ref.   Elftman, H. and Elftman, A. G., Stain Tech.,
           20 (1945), 59-62. Copyright The Williams and
           Wilkins Co.

GOMORI'S METHOD TO DEMONSTRATE CHROMAFFIN GRANULES

Fixation. 10% formalin or Bouin's fluid.

SOLUTIONS

1.   Azocarmine G solution.

      Azocarmine G   0.05 gm
      Glacial acetic acid   1 ml
      Distilled water   100 ml

2.   Aniline-alcohol.

      Aniline oil   1 ml
      95% alcohol   100 ml

3.   Phosphotungstic acid   3 gm
      Distilled water   100 ml

4.   Aniline blue solution.

      Aniline blue   0.5 gm
      Quinoline yellow (C. I. No. 47005)   2 gm
      Phosphotungstic acid   1 gm
      Distilled water   100 ml

PROCEDURE

1. Deparaffinize and hydrate sections.
2. Stain in azocarmine G solution for 60 to 90 minutes at 56 to 60°C.
3. Rinse in tap water and blot with fine filter paper.
4. Rinse in 95% alcohol.
5. Differentiate in aniline-alcohol under microscope control to the point where chromaffin cells stand out deep pink against paler cortical cells for 15 to 20 minutes.
6. Rinse briefly in tap water.
7. Place in phosphotungstic solution for 20 minutes.
8. Wash in water for 1 minute.
9. Stain in aniline blue solution for 15 to 30 minutes.
10. Rinse in tap water.
11. Dehydrate in 95% alcohol, then in absolute alcohol, two changes, 1 to 2 minutes each.
12. Clear in xylene, two changes.
13. Mount in Permount.

Results.   Chromaffin granules: purplish red. Alpha cells of pancreatic islets, some cells of the anterior pituitary, neutrophil leucocytes and myelocytes, and enterochrome cells also possess granules staining a deep purplish red to violet by this technique.

Ref.   Gomori, G., Amer. J. Clin. Path., 16 (1946), 115.

WILSON-EZRIN METHOD FOR THE HUMAN HYPOPHYSIS

Fixation. 10% formalin, Helly's fluid.

SOLUTIONS

1.   Periodic acid   0.5 gm
      Distilled water   100 ml

2.   Schiff's reagent. Bring 200 ml of distilled water to a boil, remove from flame, add 1 gm of basic fuchsin and stir until dissolved. Cool to 50°C. Filter and add 20 ml of Normal hydrochloric acid. Cool further to 25°C. Add 1 gm of sodium or potassium metabisulfite (Na2S205, K2S205). Place in the dark in a stoppered bottle for 18 to 24 hours; solution takes on an orange color. Add 0.5 gm of activated charcoal and shake well, then filter through

a coarse filter paper. Store under refrigeration in a brown stoppered bottle of the same volume. Solution is stable for several weeks. Use at room temperature.

3. Normal hydrochloric acid.

    Hydrochloric acid concentrated
    sp. gr. 1.19   83.5 ml
    Distilled water   916.5 ml

4. Sulfurous acid rinse.

    10% aqueous sodium bisulfite   6 ml
    Normal hydrochloric acid   5 ml
    Distilled water   100 ml

5. Orange G solution.

    Orange G   1 gm
    Distilled water   100 ml

6. Phosphotungstic acid   5 gm
    Distilled water   100 ml

7. Methyl blue   1 gm
    Distilled water   100 ml

8. 1% aqueous glacial acetic acid.

PROCEDURE

 1. Deparaffinize and hydrate sections.
 2. Remove mercury crystals if necessary.
 3. Rinse in distilled water.
 4. Oxidize in periodic acid solution for 5 minutes.
 5. Rinse in distilled water.
 6. Treat with Schiff reagent for 15 minutes.
 7. Rinse in three changes of sulfurous acid, 3 minutes each.
 8. Wash in running tap water for 10 minutes.
 9. Stain in Orange G for 30 seconds.
10. Mordant in phosphotungstic acid for 30 seconds.
11. Wash in running tap water for 30 seconds.
12. Stain in methyl blue for 1 minute.
13. Rinse briefly in 1% acetic acid.
14. Dehydrate in several changes of absolute alcohol.
15. Clear in xylene, two changes.
16. Mount in Permount.

Results.   PAS positive granules: red. Beta granules:
           red. Gamma granules: purple. Alpha granules
           and other acidophilic substances: orange to
           yellow.

Ref.   Wilson, W. D. and Ezrin, C., Amer. J. Path.,
           30 (1954), 891-899.

SLIDDERS' ORANGE-G-FUCHSIN-LIGHT GREEN METHOD FOR
PITUITARY CELLS

Fixation. Formol-sublimate, formol-saline, Bouin's or
           Helly's fluids.

SOLUTIONS

1.   Lendrum's celestin blue. Dissolve 5 gm of iron alum
     (ferric ammonium sulfate) at room temperature in
     100 ml of distilled water, bring to a boil, all 0.5
     gm of celestin blue, and boil for 3 minutes. Filter
     when cool and add 14 ml of glycerin. Solution lasts
     for about 1 month.

2.   Mayer's hemalum.

     Hematoxylin crystals   1 gm
     Sodium iodate   0.2 gm
     Aluminum and ammonium sulfate
     (ammonia alum)   50 gm
     Distilled water   1000 ml
     Chloral hydrate   50 gm
     Citric acid   1 gm

     Dissolve hematoxylin, sodium iodate, and the ammo-
     nia alum overnight in 1000 ml of distilled water;
     add the chloral hydrate and citric acid. Boil for
     5 minutes; when cool, it is ready for use. The
     solution keeps well.

3.   0.25% hydrochloric acid in 70% alcohol.

4.   Orange G solution.

     Orange G   0.5 gm
     95% alcohol   100 ml
     Phosphotungstic acid   2 gm

5.   Acid fuchsin solution.

    Acid fuchsin   0.5 gm
    Glacial acetic acid   0.5 ml
    Distilled water   100 ml

6.   Phosphotungstic acid   1 gm
    Distilled water   100 ml

7.   Light green solution.

    Light green SF yellowish   1.5 gm
    Glacial acetic acid   1.5 ml
    Distilled water   100 ml

PROCEDURE

1.   Deparaffinize and hydrate sections.
2.   Remove mercury crystals if necessary.
3.   Stain in celestin blue for 10 minutes.
4.   Wash well in running tap water.
5.   Stain in Mayer's hemalum for 5 minutes.
6.   Differentiate in weak acid alcohol solution for 30 seconds.
7.   Wash well in running tap water.
8.   Rinse in 95% alcohol.
9.   Stain in Orange G solution for 2 minutes.
10. Rinse in distilled water.
11. Stain in acid fuchsin solution for 2 to 5 minutes. The staining is progressive and should be continued until the basophil cells are strongly colored.
12. Rinse in distilled water.
13. Place in 1% phosphotungstic acid solution for 5 minutes.
14. Rinse in distilled water.
15. Stain in light green solution for 1 to 2 minutes.
16. Rinse in distilled water to remove excess stain.
17. Dehydrate in two changes of absolute alcohol, 1 to 2 minutes each.
18. Clear in xylene, two changes.
19. Mount in Permount.

Results.   Nuclei: black. Acidophils: orange-yellow. Basophils: magenta red. Chromophobes: pale greyish green. Erythrocytes: yellow. Stroma: green.

Ref.   Slidders, W., J. Path. Bact., 82 (1961), 532-534.

McALLISTER'S POIRRIER'S BLUE-EOSIN B. A.
PITUITARY METHOD

Fixation. Helly's fluid.

SOLUTIONS

1.   Poirrier's blue solution.

        Poirrier's blue   1 gm
        Distilled water   100 ml

2.   Eosin B. A. solution.

        Eosin B. A.*   0.4 gm
        Distilled water   100 ml

3.   Working solution.

        Poirrier's blue   15 ml
        Eosin B. A.   15 ml
        Distilled water   20 ml

PROCEDURE

1.   Deparaffinize and hydrate sections.
2.   Remove mercury crystals.
3.   Stain in working solution for 1 hour.
4.   Differentiate in absolute alcohol 2 to 3 minutes.
5.   Rinse in clean absolute alcohol.
6.   Clear in xylene, two changes.
7.   Mount in Permount.

Results. Eosinophils: red. Basophils: blue.

Ref.   Personal communication.

CROOKE-RUSSELL METHOD FOR PITUITARY GRANULES

Fixation. 10% formalin or formol-saline.

SOLUTIONS

1.   Mordant solution.

        2.5% aqueous potassium dichromate   95 ml
        Glacial acetic acid   5 ml

*Eosin B. A., ESBE Laboratory Supplies, Toronto, Ontario,
 Canada.

2.   Lugol's iodine.

      Iodine crystals   1 gm
      Potassium iodide   2 gm
      Distilled water   200 ml

      Dissolve the potassium iodide in a small amount of
      water, add iodine, and shake to dissolve. Add the
      balance of the water.

3.   Ehrlich's acid alum hematoxylin.

      Hematoxylin   4 gm
      95% alcohol   200 ml
      Distilled water   200 ml
      Glycerin   200 ml
      Aluminum and ammonium sulfate   6 gm
      Glacial acetic acid   20 ml

      Dissolve the hematoxylin in the alcohol; add re-
      maining ingredients. Expose to light and air for
      2 weeks or longer or solution may be ripened at
      once by adding 0.4 gm of sodium iodate.

4.   Acid alcohol.

      70% alcohol   99 ml
      Hydrochloric acid   1 ml

5.   Acid fuchsin solution.

      Acid fuchsin   1 gm
      Distilled water   100 ml

6.   Mallory's aniline blue-Orange G.

      Aniline blue (water soluble)   0.5 gm
      Orange G   2 gm
      1% aqueous phosphotungstic acid   100 ml

PROCEDURE

1.   Deparaffinize and hydrate sections.
2.   Place in mordant solution for 12 to 18 hours.
3.   Wash in running tap water for 10 minutes.
4.   Place in Lugol's iodine for 3 minutes.
5.   Decolorize in 95% alcohol for 1 hour.
6.   Stain in Ehrlich's acid hematoxylin for 3 to 5
      minutes.

7. Differentiate in acid alcohol.
8. Wash in running tap water until blue.
9. Stain in 1% acid fuchsin for 15 minutes.
10. Wash in running tap water for 5 minutes.
11. Rinse in distilled water.
12. Stain in aniline-blue-Orange G solution for 20 minutes.
13. Wash in running tap water for 5 minutes.
14. Differentiate in 95% alcohol for 2 to 5 minutes,
    controlling under microscope.
15. Dehydrate in absolute alcohol, two changes.
16. Clear in xylene, two changes.
17. Mount in Permount.

Results.   Acidophil granules: orange vermillion. Baso-
           phil granules: deep blue. Some of the chromo-
           phobe cells have a gray, nongranular cytoplasm;
           others contain pale gray granules, and between
           these and the ripe acidophile and basophile
           cells are transitional forms that contain gran-
           ules of intermediate shade. Connective tissue
           fibers are a bright blue; red blood cells are
           vermillion.

Ref.   Crooke, A. C. and Russell, D. S., J. Path.
           Bact., 40 (1935), 255-283.

PAGET AND ECCLESTON ALDEHYDE-THIONIN-LUXOL FAST BLUE-PAS
METHOD TO DEMONSTRATE PITUITARY GRANULES

Fixation. Saturated mercuric chloride in 10% formalin.

           Saturated aqueous mercuric chloride
           (about 7.5%)   90 ml
           40% formaldehyde   10 ml

SOLUTIONS

  1. Lugol's iodine (Langeron).

     Iodine crystals   1 gm
     Potassium iodine   2 gm
     Distilled water   200 ml

     Dissolve the potassium iodide in a small amount of
     the distilled water, add the iodine crystals, shake
     to dissolve, and add the balance of the water.

  2. Sodium thiosulfate   5 gm
     Distilled water   100 ml

3. Solution A.

Potassium permanganate	2 gm
Distilled water	100 ml

   Solution B.

Sulfuric acid	0.5 ml
Distilled water	99.5 ml

   Working solution: equal parts of solutions A and B.

4.
Potassium bisulfate	2 gm
Distilled water	100 ml

5. Aldehyde-thionin.*

Thionin (C. I. No. 52000)	0.5 gm
70% ethyl alcohol	91.5 ml
Paraldehyde	7.5 ml
Hydrochloric acid (concentrated)	1 ml

   This solution should ripen in an air-tight stoppered bottle at room temperature for 3 to 7 days before use. Effective for 10 to 14 days if kept tightly stoppered. Store in refrigerator. Use at room temperature.

6.
Luxol fast blue MBSN (Filter before use)	0.1 gm
95% alcohol	100 ml
Glacial acetic acid	0.5 ml

7.
Lithium carbonate	0.05 gm
Distilled water	100 ml

8.
Periodic acid	1 gm
Distilled water	100 ml

9. Normal hydrochloric acid.

Hydrochloric acid (concentrated, sp. gr. 1.19)	83.5 ml
Distilled water	916.5 ml

*Thionin, Chroma-Grubler, Roboz Surgical Instrument Co., Inc., Washington, D. C.

10.   Schiff's reagent. Bring 200 ml of distilled water
        to a boil, remove from flame, add 1 gm of basic
        fuchsin, and stir until dissolved. Cool to 50°C.
        Filter and add 20 ml of Normal hydrochloric acid.
        Cool further to 25°C. Add 1 gm of sodium or potas-
        sium metabisulfite (Na2S205, K2S205). Place in the
        dark in a stoppered bottle for 18 to 24 hours; solu-
        tion takes on an orange color. Add 0.5 gm of acti-
        vated charcoal and shake well, then filter through a
        coarse filter paper. Store under refrigeration in
        a brown stoppered bottle of the same volume. Solu-
        tion is stable for several weeks. Use at room tem-
        perature.

PROCEDURE

1.   Cut sections at 5 microns.
2.   Deparaffinize and hydrate sections.
3.   Remove mercury crystals.
4.   Place in equal parts of potassium permanganate and
      sulfuric acid for 2 minutes.
5.   Bleach in potassium bisulfate solution for 1 minute
      (do not use oxalic acid).
6.   Wash in water.
7.   Stain in well ripened aldehyde-thionin solution for
      10 minutes. Use a screw-capped Coplin jar.
8.   Rinse in water.
9.   Pass through 70% alcohol and 95% alcohol for a few
      seconds each.
10.   Preheat Luxol fast blue* solution to 57°C. Stain
      and maintain slides at this temperature for 30
      minutes in covered Coplin jar.
11.   Rinse in 95% alcohol.
12.   Differentiate in lithium carbonate solution.
13.   Rinse in four changes of 70% alcohol for a few
      seconds each.
14.   Wash in water.
15.   Place in periodic acid solution for 10 minutes.
16.   Place in Schiff's reagent for 30 minutes.
17.   Wash in water for 10 minutes.
18.   Dehydrate in 95% alcohol, then in absolute alcohol,
      two changes, 1 to 2 minutes each.
19.   Clear in xylene, two changes.
20.   Mount in Permount.

*Luxol fast blue, MBSN, E. I. Du Pont de Nemours & Co.,
 Organic Chemical Department, Wilmington, Delaware.

Results. The thyrotrophs are stained a dense blue-black
        by the aldehyde thionin. The granules of
        thyroidectomy cells are clearly shown.
        Gonadotrophs are easily distinguishable, since
        they are stained a clear red by the PAS
        technique, as are also the basement membranes
        of the blood vessels. Acidophils stain a clear
        intense blue-green. Chromophobes are unstained
        or very lightly stained by the luxol fast blue,
        depending on the degree to which differentiation
        has been carried out.

Ref.   Paget, G. E. and Eccleston, E.; Stain Tech.,
        35; 3 (1960), 119-122. Paget, G. E. and
        Eccleston, E.; Stain Tech., 34; (1959), 223-
        226. Copyright The Williams and Wilkins Co.

GOMORI'S CHROME ALUM HEMATOXYLIN METHOD FOR PANCREAS

Fixation. Bouin's or Helly's fluid. Place deparaffinized
         formalin-fixed tissue in Bouin's fluid for 24
         hours.

SOLUTIONS

1. Potassium permanganate   0.3 gm
    Sulfuric acid   0.3 ml
    Distilled water   100 ml

2. Sodium bisulfite   2 gm
    Distilled water   100 ml

3. 0.5N sulfuric acid.

    Sulfuric acid   27.9 ml
    Distilled water made up to   1000 ml

4. Gomori's chrome alum hematoxylin.

    1% aqueous hematoxylin   50 ml
    3% chrome alum (chromium potassium sulfate)   50 ml
    5% potassium dichromate   2 ml
    0.5N sulfuric acid   2 ml

    The solution is ripe after 24 hours and can be used
    as long as a film with a metallic sheen continues to
    form on its surface after 1 day's standing in a
    Coplin jar (about 4 to 8 weeks). Filter solution
    before use.

5. Acid alcohol.

Hydrochloric acid	1 ml
70% alcohol	99 ml

6. Phloxine solution.

Phloxine	0.5 gm
Distilled water	100 ml

7. Phosphotungstic acid solution.

Phosphotungstic acid	5 gm
Distilled water	100 ml

PROCEDURE

1. Deparaffinize and hydrate sections.
2. Remove mercury crystals.
3. Refix tissue in Bouin's fluid for 12 hours.
4. Wash thoroughly in running tap water.
5. Treat in potassium permanganate-sulfuric acid solution for 1 minute.
6. Decolorize in sodium bisulfite solution for 2 to 3 minutes.
7. Wash in tap water.
8. Stain in Gomori's chrome alum hematoxylin under microscopic control until the beta cells stand out a deep blue, 10 to 15 minutes.
9. Differentiate in acid alcohol for 1 minute.
10. Wash in tap water until the sections are clear blue.
11. Counterstain in phloxine for 5 minutes.
12. Rinse in water.
13. Immerse in phosphotungstic acid solution for 1 minute.
14. Wash in tap water for 5 minutes. The section should regain its red color.
15. Differentiate in 95% alcohol. If the sections are too red and the alpha cells do not stand out clearly, rinse the sections for about 10 to 15 seconds in 80% alcohol.
16. Dehydrate in two changes of absolute alcohol.
17. Clear in xylene, two changes.
18. Mount in Permount.

Results. Beta cells: blue. Alpha cells: red. Delta cells: pink to red and indistinguishable from alphas. Acinar granules: red to unstained in the pancreas.

Ref.   Gomori, G.; Am. J. Path., 17 (1941), 395-406.

BOWIE'S METHOD TO DEMONSTRATE JUXTAGLOMERULAR GRANULES

<u>Fixation.</u> Helly's fluid. Other fixatives may be used
but Helly's shows the most granules. Fix thin
sections (1 to 2 mm) for 24 to 48 hours. Dog
tissue for 24 hours. Small surgical and needle
biopsies less than 24 hours. In autopsy
material the J G index may not be reliable.

SOLUTIONS

1. Iodine solution.

    Iodine crystals   1 gm
    80% alcohol   100 ml

2. Sodium thiosulfate   5 gm
    Distilled water   100 ml

3. Potassium dichromate   2.5 gm
    Distilled water   100 ml

4. Bowie's solution. Dissolve 1 gm of Biebrich scarlet
    (water-soluble C. I. No. 26905) in 250 ml of distil-
    led water and 2 gm of ethyl violet (C. I. No. 42600)
    in 500 ml of distilled water.

    Filter the former through a rapid filter paper
    (Whatman No. 4) into a beaker and a little at a time
    and with constant stirring, filter the latter into
    the same beaker. The end point of neutralization is
    when a drop of the mixture placed on filter paper
    does not show scarlet color.

    Collect the precipitate of neutral dye by filtering
    and drying in an oven. To make a stock solution,
    dissolve 0.2 gm of the neutral dye in 20 ml of 95%
    alcohol. To make a working solution, add 5 drops
    of stock solution to 50 ml of 20% alcohol.

5. Differentiating solution.

    Oil of cloves* water free   50 ml
    Xylene   50 ml

* Oil Clove U. S. P., Fritzsche Brothers, Inc., N. Y.

PROCEDURE

1. Cut paraffin sections at 4 to 5 microns; avoid excess albumin in mounting.
2. Deparaffinize to 95% alcohol.
3. Place in alcoholic iodine for 3 minutes.
4. Place in sodium thiosulfate for 3 minutes.
5. Wash in running tap water for 3 minutes.
6. Mordant in 2.5% potassium dichromate 5 to 7 hours at 60°C. Allow slides to cool to room temperature.
7. Rinse well in distilled water.
8. Stain in Bowie's working solution for 15 to 16 hours at room teperature (overnight).
9. Carry the sections individually through the following steps using a Coplin jar setup. Blot section with fine filter paper.
10. Dip quickly in fresh acetone to remove excess stain but take care not to remove too much stain from the tissue. If a number of sections are being processed, change the acetone often.
11. Differentiate in fresh clove oil-xylene mixture until sections appear red or reddish purple. Sections may be rinsed in xylene and examined under microscope. Well differentiated elastic fibers in blood vessels and JG granules appear alike,-deep blue-purple. If differentiation is incomplete, return to clove oil-xylene mixture. At this point the section is cleared and, if present, the granules are visible.
12. Clear in two changes of xylene.
13. Mount in Permount.

Results. Juxtaglomerular granules, elastic fibers in blood vessels: deep blue-purple color. Tubular epithelium: Magenta.

Note.   Run a control slide known to contain JG granules to check a particular lot of dye.

Oil of clove is of use for this method only if it is water free; otherwise a milky solution will result when it is added to xylene.

Ref.   Bowie, D. J., Anat. Record, 64: (1936), 357-367.
         Pitcock, J. A., and Hartroft, P. M., Am. J.
         Path., 34 (1958), 863-884.

McNAMARA'S GIEMSA STAIN

<u>Fixation</u>. 10% formalin, Helly's fluid.

SOLUTIONS

1. Giemsa solution.

Giemsa stain* (stock solution)	10 ml
Acetone	10 ml
Methyl alcohol	10 ml
Distilled water	100 ml

2. Differentiating solution.

Colophonium (rosin, white lumps)	15 gm
Acetone	100 ml

3. Rinse solution.

Acetone	70 ml
Xylene	30 ml

PROCEDURE

1. Deparaffinize and hydrate sections.
2. Remove mercury crystals if necessary.
3. Stain in Giemsa solution for 10 to 15 minutes.
4. Rinse in tap water, check staining under microscope.
5. Differentiate in colophonium solution; control with microscope. Check for reds and pinks to appear in tissue as blue is removed. Renew solution as film forms.
6. Rinse in several changes of acetone-xylene mixture; all colophonium must be removed.
7. Without allowing the slide to dry, place in several changes of xylene.
8. Mount in Permount.

<u>Results</u>. Nuclei and bateria: blue.   Collagen and other tissue elements: pink.

<u>Ref</u>.   McNamara, W. L. J. Lab. Clin. Med., <u>18</u> (1933), 752.

*Giemsa stock solution, Gradwold Laboratory, St. Louis, Mo. Lillie formula; J. Lab. Clin. Med., 28 (1943), 15.

WOLBACH'S MODIFICATION OF THE GIEMSA STAIN

Fixation. Helly's or Zenker's fluid.

SOLUTIONS

1. Giemsa staining solution.

    Giemsa stock solution   2.5 ml
    Methyl alcohol   3 ml

    Distilled water to which has been added 2-4 drops of
    0.5% solution of sodium bicarbonate

2. Colophonium solution.

    Colophonium (rosin, white lumps)   10 gm
    Absolute alcohol   100 ml

PROCEDURE

1. Deparaffinize and hydrate sections.
2. Remove mercury crystals.
3. Pour stain over slides immediately after mixing; the
    stain should be changed twice during the first hour.
    Leave sections overnight in a third change of stain-
    ing solution.
4. Pour off stain and place sections in distilled water.
5. Differentiate slides individually under microscope
    in 95% alcohol to which a few drops of 10%
    colophonium in absolute alcohol have been added.
    (Check for reds to appear as excess blue is removed.)
6. Dehydrate sections in absolute alcohol, two changes.
7. Clear in xylene, two changes.
8. Mount in Permount.

Results. Nuclei: dark blue to violet. Collagen and
         muscle: pale pink. Rickettsiae: reddish purple.
         Erythrocytes: yellow or pink.

Ref.   Mallory, F. B., Pathological Techniques, Hafner
         Publishing Co., New York, 1968.

RALPH'S METHOD TO DEMONSTRATE HEMOGLOBIN

Fixation. Absolute alcohol, 10% formalin or Carnoy's
          fluid.

SOLUTIONS

1. Benzidine   1 gm
    Absolute methyl alcohol   100 ml

2. Hydrogen peroxide 30%   25 ml
    70% ethyl alcohol   75 ml

3. Nuclear fast red (Kernechtrot).

    Nuclear fast red   0.1 gm
    Aluminum sulfate   5 gm
    Distilled water   100 ml

    Dissolve the nuclear fast red in the aluminum sul-
    fate solution, bring to a boil, cool, and filter.
    Solution keeps well at room temperature.

PROCEDURE

 1. Deparaffinize and hydrate sections.
 2. Rinse in distilled water.
 3. Flood slide with benzidene solution for 1 minute.
 4. Drain off and flood slide with peroxide solution
    for 1 minute.
 5. Wash in distilled water for 15 seconds.
 6. Counterstain in nuclear fast red for 2 to 3 minutes.
 7. Rinse in distilled water.
 8. Dehydrate in 95% alcohol, then in absolute alcohol,
    two changes, 1 to 2 minutes each.
 9. Clear in xylene, two changes.
10. Mount in Permount.

Results. Hemoglobin: dark brown. Nuclei: red.

Ref.   Ralph, P. H.; Stain Tech., 16 (1945), 105-106.
          Copyright The Williams and Wilkins Co.

PUTT'S BENZIDINE-THIONIN METHOD TO DEMONSTRATE
HEMOGLOBIN

Fixation. 10% formalin. (Fixatives containing dichromates
          are unsuitable.)

SOLUTIONS

1. Benzidine-thionin.

Solution A		Solution B	
Thionin	0.25 gm	Benzidine	1 gm
Distilled water	100 ml	Methyl alcohol	100 ml

For use, combine equal parts of solution A and solution B and filter. The combined solution lasts for about 2 weeks.

2. Peroxide solution.

Hydrogen peroxide 30%	10 ml
Absolute alcohol	90 ml

3. Differentiating solution.

Absolute alcohol	100 ml
Glacial acetic acid	2 drops

PROCEDURE

1. Deparaffinize and hydrate sections.
2. Rinse in distilled water.
3. Stain in thionin solution for 5 minutes.
4. Carry slides individually through the peroxide solution for 1 minute and agitate gently; use slide forceps.
5. Differentiate in acetic-alcohol control under microscope.
6. Rinse quickly in absolute alcohol; this continues differentiation.
7. Clear in xylene, two changes.
8. Mount in Permount.

Results. Hemoglobin is stained an olive green if present in red blood cells or in casts in tubules of the kidneys. Hemosiderin is changed from yellow to brown. The color of hematoidin crystals and bile pigments either bilirubin or biliverdin, is unaltered. Iron in calcified vessels stains blue.

Note. Benzidien reagent (C6H4)2(N H2) or benzidine base should be used; benzidine dihydrochloride (C6H4)2(N H2) 2HCL is not suitable.

Ref. Putt, F. A. A. J. A., Arch. Path., 52 (1951), 293-294. Copyright American Medical Association.

OKAJAMA'S ALIZARIN RED S METHOD TO DEMONSTRATE
HEMOGLOBIN

Fixation.   10% formalin.

SOLUTIONS

1. 10% aqueous phosphomolybdic acid.

2. 7.7% aqueous alizarin red S.

    Working Solution

10% aqueous phosphomolybdic acid	10 ml
7.7% alizarin red S.	30 ml

3. Harris' hematoxylin.

Hematoxylin crystals	5 gm
Absolute ethyl alcohol	50 ml
Aluminum and potassium sulfate (potassium alum)	100 gm
Mercuric oxide (red)	2.5 gm
Distilled water	1000 ml

    Dissolve the hematoxylin in the alcohol and the alum
    in water with the aid of heat. Mix the two solutions
    together and bring to a boil. Withdraw the flame,
    slowly and carefully add the mercuric oxide, heat
    gently, and allow to boil for 5 minutes. Place the
    flask in cold water and cool quickly. Filter and
    add 40 ml of glacial acetic acid to improve nuclear
    staining. Filter the solution each time before use;
    solution is effective for 1 to 2 months.

PROCEDURE

1. Deparaffinize and hydrate sections.
2. Place sections in phosphomolybdic acid for 1 minute.
3. Rinse in distilled water.
4. Stain in working solution for 1 to 2 hours.
5. Wash in distilled water.
6. Wash in tap water.
7. Counterstain for 1 minute in Harris' hematoxylin.
8. Wash well in running tap water.
9. Dehydrate in 95% alcohol, then in absolute alcohol,
    two changes, 1 to 2 minutes each.
10. Clear in xylene, two changes.
11. Mount in Permount.

Results.   Hemoglobin: orange to orange red. Nuclei: blue.
             Background is reddish brown.

Ref.   Okajama, K.; Anat. Record, 11 (1916), 295.

LAIDLAW'S MODIFICATION OF BLOCK'S DOPA REACTION

Fixation.   Fresh tissue or tissue fixed in 5% formalin
             for no longer than 2 to 3 hours. Negative
             control; boiled sections. Positive control;
             human skin.

SOLUTIONS

1. Dopa solution. Dissolve 0.3 gm of 3, 4-dioxyphenyl-
    alanine (Hoffman LaRoche) in 300 ml of distilled
    water. Keep in a tightly stoppered bottle in
    refrigerator where it will remain good for many
    weeks. The solution is usable as long as it remains
    colorless; discard when it bocomes a distinct red.

2. Buffer solutions.

    Solution A
    Sodium phosphate monobasic   11 gm
    Distilled water   1000 ml

    Solution B
    Potassium hydrogen phosphate   9 gm
    Distilled water   1000 ml

3. Dopa working solution.

    Buffer solution A   2 ml
    Buffer solution B   6 ml
    Stock Dopa solution   25 ml

    Filter through fine filter paper. Should be pH 7.4.

4. Counterstain.

    Neutral red   0.5 gm
    Distilled water   100 ml

PROCEDURE

1. Cut frozen sections at 10 microns or less into
    distilled water. Do not allow sections to remain in
    distilled water for more than a few seconds as it
    weakens the reactions.

2. Transfer to buffered Dopa solution. At pH 7.4 the
   reaction will be complete at 37°C in 4 to 5 hours.
   At the end of 30 minutes examine the sections and
   change the Dopa solution. Then examine the sections
   every 30 minutes under the microscope to determine
   the proper intensity of staining. In 2 to 3 hours
   the solution turns reddish, in 3 to 4 hours a sepia
   brown. Do not allow the sections to remain in the
   solution once it becomes sepia-colored, since over-
   staining will result. A trace of alkali hastens the
   reaction; a trace of acid inhibits it. All glassware,
   therefore, must be clean.
3. Wash in distilled water.
4. Counterstain in neutral red.
5. Dehydrate in 95% alcohol, then in absolute alcohol,
   two changes, 1 to 2 minutes each.
6. Clear in xylene, two changes. Mount on slide.
7. Mount in Permount.

Results.   Sites of dopa oxidase activity: gray to black.
            Melanin retains its natural yellow-brown color.

Ref.   Laidlaw, G. F. and Blackberg, S. N.; Amer. J.
            Path., 8 (1932), 491-498.

MAXIMOW'S ALCOHOLIC THIONIN TO DEMONSTRATE MAST CELL
GRANULES

Fixation.   Absolute alcohol preferred, 10% formalin.

SOLUTIONS

1. 50% alcohol saturated with thionin about 3%.

PROCEDURE

1. Deparaffinize sections to 70% alcohol.
2. Place in alcoholic thionin for 24 to 48 hours.
3. Blot dry with fine filter paper.
4. Differentiate in two changes of 95% alcohol.
5. Dehydrate in absolute alcohol, two changes, 1 minute
   each.
6. Clear in xylene, two changes.
7. Mount in Permount.

Results.   Nuclei: blue. Mast cell granules: red to purple.

Ref.   Mallory, F. B. Pathological Technique, Hafner
            Publishing Co., New York, 1968.

ALLEN'S NEUTRAL RED METHOD TO DEMONSTRATE MAST CELLS

<u>Fixation</u>.   10% formalin.

SOLUTIONS

1.   Neutral red solution.

Neutral red	0.5 gm
50% alcohol	100 ml

2.   Mayer's hemalum.

Hematoxylin crystals	1 gm
Sodium iodate	0.2 gm
Aluminum and ammonium sulfate (ammonia alum)	50 gm
Distilled water	1000 ml
Chloral hydrate	50 gm
Citric acid	1 gm

Dissolve hematoxylin, sodium iodate and the ammonia alum overnight in 1000 ml of distilled water; add the chloral hydrate and citric acid. Boil for 5 minutes; when cool, it is ready for use. The solution keeps well.

3.   Butanol (n-Butyl alcohol)

PROCEDURE

1.   Deparaffinize and hydrate sections.
2.   Stain in Mayer's hemalum for 3 to 5 minutes.
3.   Wash in tap water until blue.
4.   Stain in neutral red solution for 10 minutes.
5.   Differentiate in 70% alcohol for 3 to 10 minutes.
6.   Dehydrate rapidly in 95% alcohol.
7.   Continue dehydration in n-butyl alcohol for 10 minutes.
8.   Clear in xylene, two changes.
9.   Mount in Permount.

<u>Results</u>.   Mast cell granules, cartilage: red. Nuclei: Blue.

<u>Ref</u>.   Allen, A. M.; Amer. J. Clin. Path., 33 (1960), 461-469.

BUNTING'S TOLUIDINE BLUE FOR METACHROMASIA

<u>Fixation</u>.   4% aqueous basic lead acetate for 2 days; Lillie's buffered formalin may also be used.

SOLUTIONS

1. Toluidine blue solution.

    Toluidine blue   0.05 gm
    Distilled water   100 ml

PROCEDURE

1. Deparaffinize and hydrate sections.
2. Rinse in distilled water.
3. Stain overnight in toluidine blue.
4. Differentiate in 95% alcohol for 2 to 3 seconds.
5. Dehydrate in absolute alcohol for 3 to 4 seconds.
6. Clear in xylene, two changes.
7. Mount in Permount.

Results.   Metachromatic material: pink. Nuclei: blue.

Note.   The basic lead acetate should be made up fresh
            just before use. Do not confuse Toluidine blue,
            C. I. No. 52040 with Toluylene blue C. I. No.
            49110.

Ref.   Personal communication.

AXURE-A METHOD FOR METACHROMATIC COMPONENTS

Fixation.   10% neutral formalin, cold absolute alcohol,
            Carnoy's, Helly's or Zenker's fluids.

SOLUTIONS

1. Azure-A solution.

    Azure-A (C. I. No. 52005)   0.01 gm
    30% alcohol   100 ml

2. 70% alcohol.

PROCEDURE

1. Deparaffinize and hydrate sections.
2. Remove mercury crystals if necessary.
3. Rinse in distilled water.
4. Stain in Azure-A solution for 5 to 10 minutes.
5. Rinse in distilled water.
6. Rinse in 70% alcohol.

7. Dehydrate in two changes of absolute alcohol, 2 to 3 minutes each.
8. Clear in xylene, two changes.
9. Mount in Permount.

Results. Metachromatic components, mucins, cartilage matrix, and mast cell granules: pink to red.

LENDRUM'S PHLOXINE-TARTRAZINE METHOD FOR INCLUSION BODIES

Fixation. Helly's, Zenker's fluids or 10% formalin.

SOLUTIONS

1. Mayer's hemalum.

   Hematoxylin crystals   1 gm
   Sodium iodate   0.2 gm
   Aluminum and ammonium sulfate (ammonia alum)   50 gm
   Distilled water   1000 ml
   Chloral hydrate   50 gm
   Citric acid   1 gm

   Dissolve hematoxylin, sodium iodate, and the ammonia alum overnight in 1000 ml of distilled water; add the chloral hydrate and citric acid. Boil for 5 minutes; when cool, it is ready for use. The solution keeps well.

2. Scott's tap water substitue.

   Sodium bicarbonate   2 gm
   Magnesium sulfate   20 gm
   Distilled water   1000 ml

3. Phloxine-calcium chloride solution.

   Phloxine B   0.5 gm
   Calcium chloride   0.5 gm
   Distilled water   100 ml

   Filter before use each time.

4. Tartrazine (Stock solution).

   Tartrazine   2 gm
   Cellosolve (ethylene glycol monoethyl ether) 100 ml

Heat in water bath to form a saturated solution.
Cool and filter.

5. Dilute tartrazine.

    Tartrizine (stock solution)   40 ml
    Cellosolve   60 ml

PROCEDURE

1. Deparaffinize and hydrate sections. (Run a control
    slide).
2. Remove mercury crystals if necessary.
3. Stain in Mayer's hemalum for 5 to 10 minutes.
4. Wash well in tap water.
5. Blue in Scott's tap water substitute for 1 to 2
    minutes.
6. Wash in tap water.
7. Place in phloxine-calcium chloride for 15 to 20
    minutes.
8. Rinse rapidly in distilled water.
9. Differentiate in stock tartrazine solution control-
    ling with microscope until the erythrocytes have
    lost the phloxine. Pour solution over slide from
    dropper bottle.
10. Rinse in tap water. This stops differentiation and
    washes out the yellow.
11. Rinse in cellosolve.
12. Stain in dilute tartrazine solution to give the
    section a canary yellow background.
13. Rinse in methyl alcohol for 1/2 to 1 minute.
14. Dehydrate in absolute alcohol.
15. Clear in xylene, two changes.
16. Mount in Permount.

Results.   Nuclei: blue. Collagen: yellow. Kurloff
            bodies in guinea pig lung, inclusions of
            infantile giant cell pneumonia, and others are
            stained red. Negri bodies: unstained.

Ref.   Lendrum, A. C.; J. Path. Bact. 59 (1947),
            399-404.

SCHILEISTEIN METHOD TO DEMONSTRATE NEGRI BODIES

Fixation. Zenker's fluid.

1. Stock solution.

    Basic fuchsin   1.8 gm
    Methylene blue   1 gm

    Glycerin   100 ml
    Methyl alcohol   100 ml

    This solution lasts indefinitely.

2. Working solution.

    Stock solution   10 drops
    Potassium hydroxide 1:40,000 aqueous   20 ml

PROCEDURE

1. Deparaffinize and hydrate sections.
2. Remove mercury crystals.
3. Rinse in distilled water.
4. Place slides on a warm hot plate, pour on stain,
    and steam for 5 minutes. Do not allow to boil.
5. Rinse in tap water.
6. Differentiate slides individually in 90% alcohol
    with gentle agitation until they take on a pale
    violet color.
7. Dehydrate in absolute alcohol.
8. Clear in xylene, two changes.
9. Mount in Permount.

Results. Negri bodies: magenta red. Nucleoli: blue-
        black. Granular inclusions: dark blue.
        Cytoplasm: blue-violet. Erythrocytes: copper.

Ref.   Schleistein, K.; Amer. J. Public Health, 27
      (1937), 1283-1285.

MANN'S METHYL BLUE-EOSIN METHOD TO DEMONSTRATE INCLUSION
BODIES

Fixation. Helly's or Zenker's fluids.

SOLUTIONS

1. Stock solutions.

    Solution A
    Eosin Y   1 gm
    Distilled water   100 ml

Solution B
Methyl blue   1 gm
Distilled water   100 ml

Working solution.

Eosin Y   6 ml
Methyl blue   6 ml
Distilled water   28 ml

2. Differentiator. Absolute alcohol containing 4 mg
    of sodium hydroxide. Add 0.1 ml of a 1% sodium
    hydroxide in alcohol to 25 ml of absolute alcohol.

3. 100 ml distilled water with 3 to 4 drops of glacial
    acetic acid.

PROCEDURE

1. Deparaffinize and hydrate sections.   (Run a control
    slide.)
2. Remove mercury crystals.
3. Stain in eosin-methyl blue solution for 24 hours at
    room temperature.
4. Wash in distilled water.
5. Differentiate in alcohol-sodium hydroxide solution.
6. Wash in absolute alcohol.
7. Wash in distilled water-acetic acid solution.
8. Dehydrate in absolute alcohol.
9. Clear in xylene.
10. Mount in Permount.

Results.   Negri bodies and erythrocytes: red. Nuclei and
              inner granules of the inclusion bodies: blue.

Ref.   Lillie, R. D.; Histopathologic Technic and
              Practical Histochemistry, 3rd., New York,
              Used with permission of McGraw-Hill, 1965.

BROWN AND BRENN METHOD TO DEMONSTRATE GRAM-POSITIVE AND
GRAM-NEGATIVE ORGANISMS IN TISSUE (MODIFIED_

Fixation.   10% formalin, Helly's fluid.

SOLUTIONS

1. Crystal violet stock solution.

Crystal violet (C. I. No. 42555)	1 gm
Distilled water	100 ml

2. Sodium bicarbonate / Distilled water

Sodium bicarbonate	5 gm
Distilled water	100 ml

3. Crystal violet working solution.

Crystal violet stock solution (filter)	1 ml
Sodium bicarbonate solution	5 drops

4. Gram's iodine.

Iodine crystals	1 gm
Potassium iodide	2 gm
Distilled water	300 ml

Dissolve the potassium iodide in 10 ml of distilled water; add iodine crystals. When dissolved, add the balance of the water.

5. Decolorizer.

Acetone	1 part
Ether	3 parts

6. Basic fuchsin stock solution / Distilled water

Basic fuchsin stock solution	0.25 gm
Distilled water	100 ml

7. Working solutions.

Basic fuchsin solution	0.1 ml
Distilled water	100 ml

8. Differentiator.

Picric acid, anhydrous	0.1 gm
Acetone	100 ml

PROCEDURE

1. Deparaffinize and hydrate sections. (Run a control slide).
2. Place slide on a staining rack* and pour on freshly prepared crystal violet working solution. Allow to stain for 2 minutes.
3. Wash in water, 1 minute.

*Southworth-Davis staining rack, Scientific Products.

4. Cover sections with Gram's iodine for 1 minute.
5. Rinse in tap water.
6. Blot section with the fine side of filter paper but do not allow to dry.
7. From a dropper bottle decolorize sections with ether-acetone solution until no more color comes off.
8. Blot but do not dry.
9. Counterstain in basic fuchsin solution for 5 minutes Iin Coplin jar).
10. Wash in water, blot but do not allow sections to dry.
11. Place in acetone briefly.
12. Decolorize with picric-acetone from a dropper bottle until the sections are yellowish pink. This is the most critical stage of the procedure and should be carried out by holding the slide over a white dish. Most of the fuchsin should be decolorized from the tissue but the Gram-negative bacteria and nuclei should remain in red.
13. Rinse in acetone (in Coplin jar).
14. Rinse in acetone-xylene, 50:50.
15. Clear in several changes of xylene.
16. Mount in Permount.

Results.   Nuclei: red. Cytoplasm: yellowish. Gram-positive bacteria: deep violet. Gram-negative bacteria: red. Basophil granules: red. Erythiocytes: yellow to red. Cartilage: pink. Striated muscle and fibrin: yellow to red.

Note.   At no time after staining with crystal violet should the section be allowed to dry. The picric acid used in the picric-acetone solution should be fresh and nearly anhydrous; otherwise a greenish rather than a yellowish background will result.

Ref.   Lillie, R. D.; Histopathologic Technic and Practical Histochemistry, 3rd ed., used with permission on McGraw-Hill, New York, 1965.

LILLIE GRAM METHOD FOR BACTERIA IN TISSUE

Fixation. 10% formalin, Helly's fluid.

SOLUTIONS

1. Crystal violet   2 gm
    95% alcohol   20 ml

2. Ammonium oxalate   1 gm
    Distilled water   100 ml

3. Working solution. When crystal violet is in
    solution add 80 ml of ammonium oxalate solution,
    mix well, and filter. Solution keeps for 2 to 3
    years. Filter before use.

4. Iodine solution (Gram-Weigert).

    Potassium iodide   2 gm
    Iodine crystals   1 gm
    Distilled water   100 ml

    Dissolve the potassium iodide in 10 ml of water.
    Add the iodine crystals. When dissolved, add the
    balance of distilled water.

5. Counterstain.

    Safranim   0.5 gm
    Distilled water   100 ml

6. Acetone   50 ml
    Xylene   50 ml

PROCEDURE

 1. Deparaffinize and hydrate sections. (Run a control
    slide.)
 2. Remove mercry crystals if necessary.
 3. Stain in crystal violet solution for 30 seconds on
    staining rack.
 4. Wash in running water for 3 to 5 minutes.
 5. Treat with iodine solution for 30 seconds.
 6. Wash in tap water 2 to 3 minutes.
 7. Rinse with acetone from a dropper bottle while slide
    is held horizontally until no more color is removed;
    10 to 15 seconds.
 8. Rinse quickly in water.
 9. Counterstain in safranin for 30 seconds.
10. Wash in water.
11. Differentiate in two changes of acetone, leaving
    cytoplasm pink and nuclei red.
12. Dehydrate in acetone-xylene 50:50.
13. Clear in xylene, two changes.
14. Mount in Permount.

Results.   Gram-positive bacteria: bluish-black. Gram-
             negative bacteria: red. Collagen, fibrin, and
             cytoplasm: pink.

Ref.   Lillie, R. D.; Arch. Path. Lab. Med., 5 (1928),
             828-834.

GLYNN'S MODIFICATION OF GRAM'S STAIN FOR GRAM-NEGATIVE
AND POSITIVE BACILLI

Fixation.   10% formalin or Helly's fluid.

SOLUTIONS

1.   Carbol-crystal-violet.

     Crystal violet   1 gm
     Phenol crystals   1 gm
     Triturate in a mortar and add
     absolute alcohol   10 ml

     Dilute this stock solution ten times with distilled
     water. Allow to stand 48 hours and filter before
     using.

2.   Gram's iodine (Gram-Weigert).

     Iodine crystals   1 gm
     Potassium iodide   2 gm
     Distilled water   100 ml

     Dissolve the potassium iodide in 10 ml of water.
     Add the iodine crystals; when dissolved, add the
     balance of distilled water.

3.   Basic fuchsin solution.

     Basic fuchsin   0.0.5 gm
     N/500 hydrochloric acid   100 ml

4.   Saturated aqueous solution of picric acid (about 1
     to 1.5%).

PROCEDURE

1.   Deparaffinize and hydrate sections. (Run a control
     slide.)
2.   Remove mercury crystals if necessary.

3.   Stain in carbol-crystal-violet solution for 2 min-
      utes on staining rack.
4.   Drain but do not wash.
5.   Apply Gram's iodine for 1 minute.
6.   Rinse in absolute acetone for 10 to 15 seconds until
      no more color is removed.
7.   Wash in running tap water for 5 minutes.
8.   Stain in basic fuchsin solution for 3 minutes.
9.   Drain but do not wash.
10.   Apply saturated picric acid solution for 3 seconds
      to 1 minute.
11.   Wash in running tap water for 5 minutes.
12.   Differentiate in absolute acetone for 10 to 15
      seconds.
13.   Clear in two changes of xylene.
14.   Mount in Permount.

Results.   Gram-positive bacteria: deep violet. Gram-
           negative bacteria: deep red. Nuclei: lighter
           red. Cytoplasm: faint yellow. Human tubercle
           bacilli are less deeply stained than other
           Gram-positive organisms and show distinct bead-
           ing. The clubs of actinomyces are red.

Note.   In using this method each slide should be
           handled individually in order to obtain satis-
           factory results. The slides should never be
           run through en masse.

Ref.   Glynn, J. H. A. M. A., Arch. Path., 20 (1935),
           896-899. Copyright American Medical Association.

GRAM-WEIGERT METHOD TO DEMONSTRATE GRAM-POSITIVE
ORGANISMS

Fixation. Zenker's fluid is preferred but 10% formalin
          or Helly's may be used.

SOLUTIONS

1.   Alum hematoxylin (Mallory).

      Hematoxylin   1 gm
      Aluminum and ammonium sulfate   20 gm
      Distilled water   400 ml
      Thymol   1 gm

      Dissolve the hematoxylin in 100 ml of distilled
      water with the aid of gentle heat; dissolve the alum
      in the rest of the water. Add thymol to prevent the

growth of mold, combine the two solutions, and allow
to ripen in a lightly stoppered flask for about 10
days. Transfer to a well stoppered brown glass
bottle. Solution is effective for 2 to 3 months.

2.   Phloxine   2.5 gm
      Distilled water   100 ml

3.   Stirling's crystal violet.

      Crystal violet   5 gm
      Absolute alcohol   10 ml
      Aniline   2 ml
      Distilled water   88 ml

      Mix the aniline oil in water, shake well, and filter.
      Dissolve the crystal violet in the alcohol; combine
      the two solutions. Solution is stable for 2 to 3
      months. Filter before use.

4.   Gram's iodine.

      Iodine crystals   1 gm
      Potassium iodide   2 gm
      Distilled water   300 ml

      Dissolve the potassium iodide in a small amount of
      water and add the iodine crystals. When dissolved,
      add the balance of distilled water.

PROCEDURE

1.   Deparaffinize and hydrate sections. (Run a control
      slide.)
2.   Remove mercury crystals if necessary.
3.   Stain lightly in alum hematoxylin.
4.   Wash well in distilled water 3 to 5 minutes.
5.   Place sections in phloxine solution for 5 to 15 min-
      utes in 60°C paraffin oven.
6.   Wash in tap water.
7.   Place slides on a staining rack and cover with Stir-
      ling's crystal violet for 10 minutes.
8.   Wash off section with Gram's iodine, pour on more,
      and allow to act for 3 minutes.
9.   Wash in water.
10.   Blot with fine filter paper and decolorize sections
      individually in several changes of aniline until
      violet clouds no longer come off. Aniline and
      xylene in equal parts may be used instead of aniline

for decolorizing organisms that stain delicately. Two to three changes of each solution should be used blotting between each change.
11. Rinse in 2 to 3 changes of xylene.
12. Mount in Permount.

Results. Gram-positive organisms: deep violet. Nuclei: blue to violet. Connective tissue: red. Gram-negative bacteria: unstained. Mycelia: blue. Clubs: pink to red.

Ref. Mallory, F. B., Pathological Technique, Hafner Publishing Co., New York, 1938.

PUTT'S METHOD TO DEMONSTRATE LEPROSY BACILLI AND ACID-FAST ORGANISMS

Fixation 10% formalin for leprosy bacilli; tubercle bacilli, any general fixative.

SOLUTIONS

1. New fuchsin solution.

   New fuchsin (magenta III C. I.
   No. 42520)   1 gm
   Carbolic acid crystals (phenol)   5 gm
   Absolute ethanol or methanol   10 ml

   Dissolve completely, gradually add while stirring distilled water to make up to 100 ml. This solution keeps for a year or more. Filter before use.

2. Saturated aqueous solution of lithium carbonate (about 2%). Solution effective for one month.

3. Differentiator.

   Glacial acetic acid   5 ml
   Absolute alcohol   95 ml

4. Counterstain.

   Methylene blue   0.5 gm
   Absolute alcohol   100 ml

PROCEDURE

1. Deparaffinize and hydrate sections. (Run a control
    slide.)
2. Remove mercury crystals if necessary.
3. Place sections in new fuchsin in Coplin jar at room
    temperature for 3 minutes.
4. Place sections in lithium carbonate for 1 minute,
    agitate sections gently. Discard lithium carbonate
    when it takes on a blue color.
5. Differentiate in acetic alcohol until sections are
    a pale pink color, 3 to 5 minutes.
6. Rinse in two changes of absolute alcohol for 2 min-
    utes each.
7. Counterstain in methylene blue for 1 to 2 minutes.
8. Decolorize in two changes of absolute alcohol; con-
    trol under microscope.
9. Clear in xylene, two changes.
10. Mount in Permount.

Results.   Acid fast bacilli: red. Hair shafts: red.
            Red corpuscles: pink. Mast cell granules: deep
            blue. Nuclei: blue. All other bacteria: blue.

Note.   This method may also be used for smears. It
            has been shown by Robboy and Vickery that ac-
            tinomyces Israelii and Nocardia asteroides may
            be demonstrated by this method.

Ref.   Putt, F. A., Amer. J. Clin. Path., 21 (1951),
            92-95.
            Robboy, S. J. and Vickery, A. L., New Eng. J.
            Med., 282 (1970), 293-296.

KINYOUN'S METHOD FOR ACID-FAST ORGANISMS

Fixation. 10% formalin, Helly's fluid.

SOLUTIONS

1. Harris' hematoxylin.

Hematoxylin crystals	5 gm
Absolute ethyl alcohol	50 ml
Aluminum and potassium sulfate	
(potassium alum)	100 gm
Mercuric oxide (red)	2.5 gm
Distilled water	1000 ml

Dissolve the hematoxylin in the alcohol and the alum in water with the aid of heat. Mix the two solutions together and bring to a boil. Withdraw the flame, slowly and carefully add the mercuric oxide, heat gently, and allow to boil for 5 minutes. Place the flask in cold water and cool quickly. Filter and add 40 ml of glacial acetic acid to improve nuclear staining. Filter the solution each time before use; solution is effective for 1 to 2 months.

2.   Carbol-fuchsin solution.

Basic fuchsin	4 gm
95% alcohol	20 ml
Melted carbolic acid crystals	8 ml
Distilled water	100 ml

Combine ingredients; heat to dissolve. Then add water and filter before use.

3.   70% alcohol   99 ml
      Concentrated hydrochloric acid   1 ml

PROCEDURE

1.   Deparaffinize and hydrate sections. (Run a control slide.)
2.   Remove mercury crystals if necessary.
3.   Stain in Harris' hematoxylin for 5 minutes.
4.   Wash in running tap water until blue.
5.   Place sections in carbol-fuchsin at 37°C for 1 hour.
6.   Decolorize in acid alcohol for 2 to 3 minutes.
7.   Rinse in 95% alcohol, then in absolute alcohol, two changes, 1 to 2 minutes each.
8.   Clear in xylene, two changes.
9.   Mount in Permount.

Results. Acid-fast organisms: red. Nuclei: blue.

Ref.   Kinyoun, J. J., Amer. J. Public Health, 5 (1915), 867-870.

SPENGLER'S METHOD TO DEMONSTRATE ACID-FAST ORGANISMS

Fixation. 10% formalin or heat-fixed smears.

SOLUTIONS

1.   New fuchsin solution.

New fuchsin C. I. No. 42520	1 gm
Phenol crystals	5 gm
Absolute alcohol	10 ml

Dissolve the fuchsin in the alcohol-phenol, gradually add while shaking distilled water to bring
the volume up to 100 ml. This solution keeps for a
year or more. Filter before use.

2.   Picric acid-alcohol.

| Picric acid | 2 gm |
| Distilled water | 40 ml |

Let stand for 24 hours, filter, and add an equal
volume of 95% alcohol.

3.   Nitric acid solution.

| Nitric acid | 15 ml |
| Distilled water | 85 ml |

PROCEDURE

1.   Deparaffinize and hydrate sections. (Run a control
     slide.)
2.   Place sections in fuchsin solution at room tempera-
     ture for 3 to 5 minutes.
3.   Drain the fuchsin solution and rinse in picric acid-
     alcohol for 2 to 3 seconds.
4.   Apply 3 to 4 drops of nitric acid solution for 5
     seconds.
5.   Pour off the nitric acid and apply the picric acid-
     alcohol solution again until the preparation appears
     yellow.
6.   Wash in 95% alcohol for 1 minute.
7.   Smears may be left to dry. Sections may be quickly
     rinsed in absolute alcohol, cleared in xylene, and
     mounted in Permount.

Results.   Acid-fast organisms stain black on a yellowish
           background.

Note.   This method claims to be useful for people
        suffering from color blindness, however, it may
        prove confusing in tissue containing other pig-
        ments.

Ref.   Gray, Peter, The Microtomists Formulary and
              Guide, Constable & Co., Ltd., 1954, p. 478.

ZIEHL-NEELSEN METHOD TO DEMONSTRATE TUBERCLE BACILLI

Fixation. 10% formalin, Helly or Zenker's fluids.

SOLUTIONS

1.   Harris' hematoxylin.

      Hematoxylin crystals   5 gm
      Absolute ethyl alcohol   50 ml
      Aluminum and potassium sulfate
      (potassium alum)   100 gm
      Mercuric oxide (red)   2.5 gm
      Distilled water   1000 ml

      Dissolve the hematoxylin in the alcohol and the
      alum in water with the aid of heat. Mix the two
      solutions together and bring to a boil. Withdraw
      the flame, slowly and carefully add the mercuric
      oxide, heat gently, and allow to boil for 5 minutes.
      Place the flask in cold water and cool quickly.
      Filter and add 40 ml of glacial acetic acid to im-
      prove nuclear staining. Filter the solution each
      time before use; solution is effective for 1 to 2
      months.

2.   Verhoeff's carbol-fuchsin.

      Basic fuchsin   2 gm
      Absolute alcohol   50 ml
      Melted carbolic acid crystals   25 ml

      Combine the ingredients, leave overnight in 60°C
      oven, cool, and filter. This solution keeps well
      and does not require further filtration before use.

3.   Acid alcohol.

      70% alcohol   99 ml
      Hydrochloric acid   1 ml

PROCEDURE

   1. Deparaffinize and hydrate sections. (Run a control
      slide.)
   2. Remove mercury crystals if necessary.

3. Stain in Harris hematoxylin for 5 minutes.
4. Wash well in tap water until section is blue.
5. Stain in Verhoeff's carbol-fuchsin in 60°C oven for 1 hour in a covered dish, or overnight at room temperature.
6. Decolorize in acid alcohol until section is pale pink.
7. Wash well in tap water to which has been added 2 to 3 drops of 28% ammonium hydroxide per 200 ml.
8. Dehydrate in 95% alcohol, then in absolute alcohol, two changes, 1 to 2 minutes each.
9. Clear in xylene, two changes.
10. Mount in Permount.

Results. Turbercle bacilli: red. Nuclei: blue.

Ref.   Mallory, F. B., Pathological Technique, Hafner Publishing Co., New York, 1968.

CARBOL-FUCHSIN-AURAMINE PHENOL METHOD TO DEMONSTRATE TUBERCLE BACILLI

Fixation. 10% formalin, Helly's fluid.

SOLUTIONS

1.   Carbol-fuchsin.

     Basic fuchsin   1 gm
     Phenol (carbolic acid)   5 gm
     Alcohol   10 ml
     Distilled water   100 ml

     Dissolve the fuchsin in the alcohol and the phenol in water; mix the two solutions. Add water and filter.

2.   Auramine-phenol.

     3% aqueous phenol   100 ml
     Auramine-O (C. I. No. 43815)   0.3 gm

     Shake well and filter.

3.   Acid alcohol.

     70% alcohol   99 ml
     Hydrochloric acid   1 ml

PROCEDURE

1. Deparaffinize and hydrate sections. (Run a control slide.)
2. Remove mercury crystals if necessary.
3. Place in hot filtered carbol-fuchsin solution for 2 to 5 minutes.
4. Wash in water.
5. Decolorize in acid alcohol for 5 minutes.
6. Wash in water.
7. Counterstain in auramine-phenol for 5 minutes.
8. Wash in water.
9. Dehydrate rapidly in 95% alcohol, then in absolute alcohol, two changes.
10. Clear in xylene, two changes.
11. Mount in Permount.

Results. Tubercle bacilli: red. Background: yellow.

Ref.   Andrla, O. J., Gazette Med. Lab. Tech., 3 (1955).

BERG'S METHOD TO DEMONSTRATE SPERMATOZOA IN TISSUE SECTIONS

Fixation. 10% formalin, Helly's fluid.

SOLUTIONS

1. Putt's carbol-fuchsin.

    New fuchsin   1 gm
    Phenol crystals   5 gm
    Absolute alcohol   10 ml
    Distilled water to bring the volume
    up to   100 ml

    Dissolve fuchsin and phenol in alcohol, gradually add while agitating the distilled water. Filter before use.

2. Saturated aqueous solution of lithium carbonate (about 2%).

3. Decolorizer.

    Glacial acetic acid   5 ml
    Absolute alcohol   100 ml

4.   Methylene blue counterstain.

     Methylene blue   0.5 gm
     Absolute alcohol   100 ml

PROCEDURE

1.   Deparaffinize and hydrate sections.
2.   Remove mercury crystals if necessary.
3.   Rinse in distilled water.
4.   Stain in carbol-fuchsin solution for 3 minutes.
5.   Place directly in lithium carbonate solution for 1
     minute; discard solution.
6.   Decolorize in acetic-alcohol for 5 minutes. Agitate
     slide.
7.   Rinse in two changes of absolute alcohol for 1 min-
     ute each.
8.   Counterstain in methylene blue for 30 to 60 seconds.
9.   Rinse rapidly in two changes of absolute alcohol.
10. Clear in xylene, two changes.
11. Mount in Permount.

Results. Spermatozoa: brilliant red. Erythrocytes:
          pink. Other tissue elements: blue.

Ref.   Berg, J. W., Amer. J. Clin. Path., 23 (1953),
          5, 513-515.

GROCOTT'S METHENAMINE SILVER METHOD TO DEMONSTRATE FUNGI

Fixation. 10% formalin, Helly's fluid.

SOLUTIONS

1.   Oxidizer.

     Chromic acid   5 gm
     Distilled water   100 ml

2.   Sodium bisulfite   1 gm
     Distilled water   100 ml

3.   Silver nitrate   5 gm
     Distilled water   100 ml

4.   Methenamine*   3 gm
     Distilled water   100 ml

*Methenamine (hexamethylene tetramine), Fisher Scientific
 Co.

5.   Borax (sodium borate)   5 gm
        Distilled water   100 ml

6.   Stock Methenamine silver solution.

        Methenamine 3%   100 ml
        Silver nitrate 5%   5 ml

        A white precipitate appears but dissolves on shaking.
        The clear solution lasts for months if kept refrig-
        erated.

7.   Working solution of Methenamine silver.

        Borax 5%   2 ml
        Distilled water   25 ml
        Stock solution of Methenamine silver   25 ml

8.   Toning solution.

        1:500 aqueous yellow gold chloride.

9.   Sodium thiosulfate   2 gm
        Distilled water   100 ml

10.   Nuclear fast red (Kernechtrot) counterstain.

        Nuclear fast red   0.1 gm
        Aluminum sulfate   5 gm
        Distilled water   100 ml

        Dissolve the nuclear fast red in the aluminum sul-
        fate solution, bring to a boil, cool, and filter.
        Solution keeps well at room temperature.

11.   Stock light green solution.

        Light green S. F. Yellowish   0.2 gm
        Distilled water   100 ml
        Glacial acetic acid   0.2 gm

12.   Working solution.

        Stock light green solution   10 ml
        Distilled water   100 ml

PROCEDURE

1. Deparaffinize and hydrate sections. (Run a control
    slide.)
2. Remove mercury crystals if necessary.
3. Oxidize sections in 5% chromic acid for 1 hour.
4. Wash in running tap water for 5 minutes.
5. Rinse sections in 1% sodium bisulfite for 1 minute.
6. Wash in tap water for 5 minutes.
7. Rinse in three changes of distilled water.
8. Place sections in Methenamine silver working solu-
    tion at 45 to 50°C for 1 hour, or until sections
    turn a light brown. Sections may be rinsed in dis-
    tilled water and examined under microscope. Fungi
    should appear dark brown; overstaining will cause
    connective tissue to stain. Do not use metallic
    forceps in silver solution.
9. Rinse in 3 to 4 changes of distilled water.
10. Tone in yellow gold chloride for 5 minutes.
11. Rinse in distilled water.
12. Fix in 2% sodium thiosulfate for 5 minutes.
13. Wash in tap water.
14. Stain nuclei in nuclear fast red (Kernechtrot) for
    10 minutes.
15. Rinse in tap water.
16. Counterstain in light green for 30 seconds.
17. Dehydrate in 95% alcohol, then in absolute alcohol,
    two changes, 1 to 2 minutes each.
18. Clear in xylene, two changes.
19. Mount in Permount.

Results. Fungi are sharply delineated in black with the
          inner parts of mycelia and hyphae stained an
          old rose as a result of the gold toning. Mucin
          also assumes a rose-red color. Our modifica-
          tion at step 14 stains nuclei red.

          Mowry's modification. Instead of chromic acid,
          0.5 gm of periodic acid in 100 ml of distilled
          water gives a stronger and more consistent
          staining. Sections may also be counterstained
          with hematoxylin and eosin if tissue detail is
          important.

Note.   All glassware should be chemically clean.

Ref.   Grocott, R. G., Amer. J. Clin. Path., 25 (1955),
          975-979.

GRIDLEY'S METHOD TO DEMONSTRATE FUNGI

Fixation. 10% formalin, Helly's or Zenker's fluid.

SOLUTIONS

1.   Chromic acid solution.

      Chromic acid   4 gm
      Distilled water   100 ml

2.   Schiff reagent. Bring 200 ml of distilled water to
      a boil, remove from flame, and add 1 gm of basic
      fuchsin and stir until dissolved. Cool to 50°C.
      Filter and add 20 ml of Normal hydrochloric acid.
      Cool further to 25°C. Add 1 gm of sodium or potas-
      sium metabisulfite (Na2S205, K2S205). Place in the
      dark in a stoppered bottle for 18 to 24 hours; solu-
      tion takes on an orange color. Add 0.5 gm of acti-
      vated charcoal and shake well, then filter through a
      coarse filter paper. Store under refrigeration in
      a brown stoppered bottle of the same volume. Solu-
      tion is stable for several weeks. Use at room tem-
      perature.

3.   Normal hydrochloric acid.

      Concentrated hydrochloric acid, sp.
      gr. 1.19   83.5 ml
      Distilled water   916.5 ml

4.   Sodium metabisulfite solution.

      Sodium metabisulfite (NA2S205)   10 gm
      Distilled water   100 ml

5.   Sulfurous acid rinse.

      Sodium metabisulfite 10%   6 ml
      Normal hydrochloric acid   5 ml
      Distilled water   100 ml

6.   Aldehyde-fuchsin solution (Gomori).

      Basic fuchsin   1 gm
      Alcohol 70%   200 ml
      Paraldehyde   2 ml
      Concentrated hydrochloric acid   2 ml

Let stand at room temperature for 3 days until solution turns deep purple. Keep in refrigerator. Filter and allow to reach room temperature before using.

7.   Metanil yellow solution.

Metanil yellow	0.25 gm
Distilled water	100 ml
Glacial acetic acid	2 drops

PROCEDURE

1. Deparaffinize and hydrate sections. (Run a control slide.)
2. Remove mercury crystals if necessary.
3. Oxidize in chromic acid for 1 hour.
4. Wash in running tap water for 5 minutes.
5. Place in Schiff's reagent for 15 minutes.
6. Rinse in three changes of sulfurous acid rinse, 2 minutes each.
7. Wash for 15 minutes in running tap water.
8. Rinse in several changes of 70% alcohol.
9. Place slides in aldehyde-fuchsin solution for 15 to 30 minutes.
10. Rinse off excess stain with two or three changes of 95% alcohol.
11. Rinse in tap water.
12. Counterstain lightly in metanil yellow for about 1 minute.
13. Rinse in water.
14. Dehydrate in 95% alcohol, then in absolute alcohol, two changes, 1 to 2 minutes each.
15. Clear in xylene, two changes.
16. Mount in Permount.

Results. Mycelia: deep blue. Background: yellow. Elastic tissue and mucin also stain a deep blue.

Ref.   Gridley, M. F., Amer. J. Clin. Path., 23 (1953), 303-307.

WARTHIN STARRY METHOD FOR SPIROCHETES IN SECTIONS: MODIFIED

Fixation. 10% formol-saline.

SOLUTIONS

1.   Acetate buffer.

      Solution A
      Sodium acetate   16.4 gm
      Distilled water   1000 ml

      Solution B
      Glacial acetic acid   11.8 ml
      Distilled water   1000 ml

2.   Working buffer solution: pH 3.6.

      Sodium acetate   1.5 ml
      Glacial acetic acid   18.5 ml
      Distilled water   480 ml

3.   Silver solution.

      Silver nitrate   1 gm
      Acetate buffer   100 ml

4.   Reducing solution: prepare just before use.

      Silver nitrate 2%   15 ml
      Gelatin   37.5 ml
      Hydroquinone 0.15%   20 ml

      The solutions above should all be made up with ace-
      tate buffer.

PROCEDURE

1.   Deparaffinize sections and hydrate to acetate buffer.
      Leave for 10 minutes.
2.   Place in silver solution for 1 hour at 55°C in
      covered Coplin jar.
3.   Place sections in freshly prepared reducing solution
      preheated to 55°C for 3 to 5 minutes; sections turn
      a golden brown color.
4.   Pour off reducing solution and wash several times
      with heated 55°C tap water, then with acetate buffer.
5.   Dehydrate in 95% alcohol then in absolute alcohol,
      two changes, 1 to 2 minutes each.
6.   Clear in xylene, two changes.
7.   Mount in Permount.

Results.   Spirochetes: black.   Tissue elements: pale
           yellowish brown.

Note.   Only glass distilled water should be used.
             Glassware should be chemically clean.

Ref.   Carleton's Histological Technique, 4ED Drury,
             R. A. D. and Wallington, E.A. (Ed.) Oxford
             University Press. London, England.

LEVADITI'S BLOCK METHOD TO DEMONSTRATE SPIROCHETES

Fixation. Tissue blocks should be cut about 1 mm thick
          and fixed in 10% formalin for 1 to 4 days at
          room temperature.

SOLUTIONS

1.   Silver solution.

      Silver nitrate   2 gm
      Distilled water   100 ml

2.   Reducing solution.

      Pyrogallic acid   4 gm
      Formaldehyde 40%   5 ml
      Distilled water   100 ml

PROCEDURE

 1.   Rinse blocks of tissue in tap water, then place in
      95% alcohol for 24 hours.
 2.   Place in distilled water until blocks sink to bottom
      of container.
 3.   Place tissue in the silver nitrate solution in a
      chemically clean brown bottle and keep in 37°C oven
      in the dark for 2 to 5 days, changing the solution
      daily.
 4.   Rinse in several changes of distilled water.
 5.   Reduce in pyrogallic acid solution at room tempera-
      ture for 24 to 72 hours in the dark.
 6.   Wash well in distilled water.
 7.   Dehydrate in 80%, 95%, and absolute alcohol.
 8.   Clear in toluene.
 9.   Infiltrate tissue with paraffin in vacuum oven, two
      or three changes of paraffin, 30 minutes each.
10.   Embed in fresh paraffin.
11.   Cut sections at 5 microns, mount on slides, and
      place in oven to dry.
12.   Remove paraffin with xylene and mount in Permount.

Results.   Spirochetes: black. Background: yellow.

Note.   Because penetration is sometimes uneven a num-
            ber of sections should be cut and mounted on
            slides; the 24 to 72 hour reduction time per-
            mits tissue blocks to be removed at intervals,
            one of which should yield satisfactory results.
            All glassware should be chemically clean. Use
            large volumes of silver solution at least 20
            to 1.

Ref.   Levaditi, C. and Manouelian; Ct. Rd., So. Biol.
            60 (1906), 134-136.

CAMPBELL AND ROSAHN METHOD TO DEMONSTRATE SPIROCHETES

Fixation. 10% buffered formalin. Fix tissue blocks, 2
          to 5 mm in thickness, for 12 to 24 hours.

SOLUTIONS

1.   Silver nitrate   3 gm
      50% ethyl alcohol   100 ml

2.   Developer solution. Filter before use. Prepare
      fresh for each group of tissue.

      Photoglycerin*   0.5 gm
      Sodium sulfite   0.5 gm
      50% ethyl alcohol   100 ml

3.   Potassium ferricyanide (prepare fresh)   1.5 gm
      Distilled water   100 ml

PROCEDURE

   1. Wash tissue in three changes of distilled water for
       30 minutes.
   2. Place in 95% methyl alcohol for 12 to 24 hours.
   3. Place tissue in silver nitrate solution in a chem-
       ically clean amber bottle, in 37°C oven for 12 to
       24 hours.
   4. Leave in amber bottle and wash in three changes of
       distilled water.

*Photoglycerin (P-Hydroxyphenyl) glycine, Fisher Scien-
 tific Co.

5. Transfer to developer solution in brown bottle for 12 to 24 hours at room temperature.
6. Wash in three changes of distilled water for 1 hour.
7. Dehydrate tissue blocks in 80% alcohol (2 hours), 95% alcohol (2 hours), absolute alcohol (2 hours), aniline oil (1 hour or until blocks become transparent and sink), xylene, three changes (1 hour each). Infiltrate in paraffin in vacuum oven in two changes of paraffin 1 hour each. Embed.
8. Cut sections at 5 microns and mount on albuminized slides. Dry in oven as usual.
9. Deparaffinize and hydrate sections.
10. Cover sections with potassium ferricyanide solution. (The section changes from gray-green to colorless or cloudy white within 1 to 2 minutes. Slight prolongation of time does not change the apparent silver content of the spirochetal form.)
11. Wash in three changes of distilled water for 1 to 2 hours.
12. Dehydrate in 95% alcohol, then in absolute alcohol, two changes, 1 to 2 minutes each.
13. Clear in xylene, two changes.
14. Mount in Permount.

Results. Spirochetes and spirochetal forms appear blue-black against a colorless background.

Ref. Campbell, R. E. and Rosahn, P. D., Yale J. Biol. Med., 22 (1950), 6, 527-543.

Chapter 12

NEUROPATHOLOGICAL METHODS

The various delicate tissue elements of which the central
nervous system is composed sets it apart from other organs.
Because of the lack of connective tissue exept in the
meninges, brain and spinal cord are relatively soft in
the fresh state when compared to other organs. This is
especially noticeable in infant brain which retains a
gelatinous consistency even after prolonged fixation in
formalin.

Brain

Autolytic changes take place rapidly in the central nervous system. As stated by Lillie, "The practice of hardening of entire human brain without perfusion, by immersion in dilute formaldehyde solution or other fixatives,
before dissection, can only be condemmed." Brains obtained
at autopsy after embalming with solutions that usually
contain formaldehyde in varying amounts should be processed as unfixed tissue. If the pressure used in this
procedure is excessive, a cerebellar pressure cone can
develop; vacuoles may also be present around neurons in
stained sections.
     The following method is suggested to perfuse brain
obtained at autopsy.

1.   Carefully remove brain, weigh, and place immediately
     in Ringer's solution.

     Concentrated Ringer's solution

     Sodium chloride   56 gm
     Potassium chloride   3 gm
     Calcuim chloride   2 gm
     Distilled water   500 ml

For use dilute 200 ml of Ringer's solution with 4000 ml of
distilled water.

2.   Tie cannula in one vertebral artery and tie off both
     internal carotids and the other vertebral artery.
     Leave threads long enough to suspend brain.
3.   Clear vascular system using 300 to 500 ml of slowly
     injected atmospheric air or 500 to 1000 ml of Ring-
     er's solution.
4.   Fix by gravity injection of approximately 1 ml of
     10% formalin for each gram weight of brain.
5.   Suspend brain in 10% formalin, to prevent flattening.
6.   If fixation by injection is good, sections may be
     taken on the fifth day. If injection is poor, the
     formalin should be changed daily for the first
     three days, then every two days for the next week.

Spinal Cord

1.   In removing and subsequent handling of unfixed
     spinal cord, great care should be taken not to kink,
     stretch, or compress it. Swank and Davenport have
     demonstrated with the Marchi method that artifically
     induced trauma may show up as blackened areas of
     myelin in otherwise normal cord.
2.   To suspend in the fixative, open the dura posteriorly
     and attach to a wooden board with thumbtacks through
     the dura. Place in a tall jar or cylinder in 10%
     formalin.
3.   Remove from board and cut out blocks after 24 to 28
     hours.

Representative blocks of surgical material should be
placed in Cajal's formalin-ammonium-bromide and 10% formalin.

Staining Techniques

Frozen, paraffin, and celloidin processed materials are
all applicable to tissue of the central nervous system,
any one of which may be necessary to demonstrate a
specific tissue component. Many routing staining techniques are applicable to neuropatnological material processed by the paraffin method. Mallory's phosphotungstic
acid hematozylin will demonstrate astrocytes and their
expansions. Nerve fibers, myelin, and Nissl granules
can be shown be specific methods. Hematoxylin and eosin
will reveal only the nuclei of neuroglia cells.
     Because of the density and high lipid content of
neurological material, dehydration, clearing, and infiltration must be increased and vacuum infiltration is recommended. Overheating in paraffin during infiltration

and embedding will result in minute fragmentation of
tissue; excessive cooling with ice when sectioning will
result in the same artifact.

Dehydration Schedule for Brain Sections

The tissue processor is set to change every four
hours as follows:

95% alcohol	three changes
Absolute alcohol	three changes
Absolute and xylene 50/50	two changes
Xylene	three changes

Tissue is infiltrated with Paraplast in vacuum oven,
three changes, 2 hours each.

A well sharpened microtome knife is a must, serrations
rations show up prominently in brain and spinal cord
even though in some cases thicker sections are necessary.
To avoid loss of sections during staining, Masson's
gelatin water method of affixing sections using a slide
warmer is preferable.

Frozen sections are necessary for certain specialized metallic techniques to allow detail study of various
neuroglia cells and their expansions, such as oligodend
roglia, microglia, and fibrous and protoplasmic astrocytes originally described by Cajal and Hortega. Many
require special fixatives which should be prepared in
advance. These highly specialized and somewhat empirical
methods are not usually carried out in a routine histology
laboratory and present a challenge even to a well trained
technologist; however, when successful the results are
so rewarding that every effort is worthwhile.

Metallic methods used to demonstrate tissue elements
of the central nervous system depend upon the use of
various silver carbonate, ammoniacal silver nitrate, and
gold sublimate solutions, many of which are quite involved. They are not true dying procedures, but impregnation
or precipitation methods in which metallic silver or
gold is deposited on the various tissue elements and
made visible by reduction comparable to photographic
procedure.

The deposit should be as fine as possible, not
coarse or granular in appearance, and if successful will
appear as a well stained section. Because metallic impregnation methods are so capricious, it is well to carry
through a number of sections, varying the time for their
immersion is silver and in reducing solutions. Since it

is not always possible to obtain consistent results on
various tissue elements, a record should be kept of
modifications introduced for a given method.

Petri and glass-covered Stender or crystalizing
dishes are convenient glassware in which to carry free
frozen sections through the various solutions. Silver
carbonate or ammoniacal silver nitrate solutions should
be kept covered during the staining procedure; otherwise
a metallic dross will form on the surface, especially if
the solution is heated.

Certain precautions must be taken to avoid extraneous
precipitates. A set of glassware should be reserved for
these methods and chemically cleaned as follows:

1.   Rinse in water.
2.   Place in glassware-cleaning solution overnight.

Potassium dichromate   215 gm
Water   2400 ml
Sulfuric acid   400 ml

Dissolve the dichromate in water and slowly and carefully
add the sulfuric acid; allow to cool. The solution
should always be made up in Pyrex glassware.

3.   Wash in running tap water overnight.
4.   Wash well with a good detergent.
5.   Wash well in running tap water.
6.   Rinse in distilled water before use.

SOLUTIONS

A.   Distilled water used to prepare metallic solutions
      should be glass-distilled, fresh, and of the highest
      purity.
B.   All silver solutions should be filtered through a
      Whatman No. 1 filter paper before use. If the
      solution can be used again, refilter it back into
      the bottle.
C.   Stock solutions should be kept in chemically clean
      brown glass stoppered bottles.
D.   Glass "hockey sticks" should be used to transfer
      frozen sections through the various silver and gold
      solutions and rinsed in distilled water as tissue is
      transfered from one solution to another. Metallic
      instruments should be avoided.
E.   All chemicals should be of the highest purity.

Dehydration and Mounting

A rapid method to dehydrate, clear, and mount loose sections without shrinkage, folds or wrinkles, which
usually occur when unmounted sections are carried through
the dehydration and clearing sequence is given below.

    With the aid of a dissection needle, carefully
mount a section on a slide from the last wash water, making
certain that the section is free from folds. This is
best carried out against a white background. Holding the
section in place on the slide with the needle, drain off
excess water. Place the slide with the section side up
between 5 to 6 sheets of Whatman No. 1 filter paper,
folded in half, the fine side next to the sections. With
gentle pressure blot the section by running the index
finger back and forth over the slide; discard the inner
layers of paper as they become wet.

    Holding the slide horizontally at a slight angle
over a waste jar, carefully pour absolute alcohol over
the section from a droper bottle for about 30 seconds;
repeat procedure with carbol-creosote-xylene and finally
with pure xylene until clear. Mount in Permount.

    If silver impregnated sections are overstained, 4%
aqueous glacial acetic acid may be used to reduce the
silver to the desired intensity. After gold toinng
sections that are too light may be intensified by treatment with 4% aqueous oxalic acid which reduces the gold.
The sections takes on a purplish tinge and fibers seem to
stand out more prominently.

    Wallington points to the explosive properties of
annomiacal-silver solutions caused by formations of silver
fulminate, silver nitride, and silver azide. He cautions
that (1) silver solutions should not be prepared in the
laboratory in the presence of formalin fumes; (2)
chemically clean glassware should be used; (3) solutions
should not be exposed to sunlight, especially if the
container is silvered. Ammoniacal-silver solutions
should be treated with a dilute hydrochloric acid or a
solution of sodium chloride before being discarded.

Ref.   Wallington, E. A., J. Med. Lab. Tech., 22 (1965)

CAJAL'S URANUIM SILVER METHOD TO DEMONSTRATE THE GOLGI
APPARATUS

Fixation.   Place 2 to 3-mm thick tissue in the follow-
             ing solution for 8 to 24 hours. It is best to
             use 3 to 4 pieces of tissue, and vary the time
             of fixation and silvering.

Best results are obtained in young (20-day) dog, cat, or rabbit tissue.

Uranyl nitrate	1 gm
Distilled water	85 ml
Formaldehyde	15 ml

SOLUTIONS

1. Silver solution: prepare fresh.

Silver nitrate	2 gm
Distilled water	100 ml

2. Cajal's developer: prepare fresh; solution darkens with age.

Hydroquinone	2 gm
Formaldehyde 40%	15 ml
Distilled water	100 ml
Anhydrous sodium sulfate	0.15 gm

3. Toning solution

    1:500 yellow gold chloride.

PROCEDURE

1. Wash blocks quickly in distilled water.
2. Place blocks in 2% silver nitrate solution for 2 to 3 days in the dark at room temperature. Change twice during impregnation. Use a chemically clean brown glass jar.
3. Wash quickly in distilled water.
4. Reduce in hydroquinone solution for 8 to 12 hours.
5. Wash blocks in distilled water.
6. Dehydrate rapidly, especially in absolute alchol, and embed in paraffin.
7. Cut sections at 6 to 7 microns, mount, and dry in oven as usual.
8. Deparaffinize sections and hydrate to distilled water.
9. Tone in yellow gold chloride for 5 to 10 minutes.
10. Wash in distilled water.
11. Dehydrate in 95% alcohol, then in absolute alcohol, two changes, 1 to 2 minutes each.
12. Clear in xylene, two changes.
13. Mount in Permount.

Penfield's modification. After step 10, stain in dilute Unna's polychrome methylene blue, rinse through graded alcohols to absolute and clear as usual.

Unna's polychrome methylene blue
Methylene blue   1 gm
Distilled water   100 ml
95% alcohol   20 ml
Potassium carbonate   1 gm

Boil down to 100 ml on a water bath.

Results.   Golgi apparatus: black. Secondary nuclear
            staining allows study and differentiation of
            other types of cells.

Note.   All glassware should be chemically clean and
            glass stoppered to aviod precipitates.

Ref.   Cajal Ramon Y.; Trav. Del Lab. Inves. Biol.
            Univ. Madrid., 10 (1912), 209-220.

DA FANO'S COBALT SILVER METHOD TO DEMONSTRATE THE GOLGI
APPARATUS

Fixation.   For delicate tissue and embryos, reduce the
            amount of formalin to prevent shrinkage. Fix
            small pieces of tissue 2 to 4 mm thick for 3
            to 4 hours. For adult tissue increase the
            formalin to 15 ml. Fix normal adult tissue 5
            to 8 hours; spinal cord and brain for 10 to 18
            hours. Run 3 to 4 tissues and vary fixation.

Fixative.   Cobalt nitrate   1 gm
            Distilled water   100 ml
            Fresh formaldehyde 40%   6-15 ml

Add formaldehyde just before use.

SOLUTIONS

1.   Silver solution: prepare fresh.

      Silver nitrate   1.5-2 gm
      Distilled water   100 ml

Use 2% solution for brain and spinal cord and fatty
tissue.

2.   Cajal's developer: prepare fresh; solution darkens
      with age.

      Hydroquinone   2 gm
      Formaldehyde 40%   6 ml
      Distilled water   100 ml
      Anhydrous sodium sulfite   0.5 gm

3.   Toning solution.

Solution A
Sodium thiosulfate   3 gm
Ammonium sulphocyanide   3 gm
Distilled water   100 ml

Solution B
Yellow gold chloride   1 gm
Distilled water   100 ml

Mix equal parts of A and B just before use. Separate
solutions keep well.

PROCEDURE

1. Rinse blocks in distilled water, 30 seconds.
2. Impregnate blocks in silver nitrate solution for
    36 to 48 hours at room temperature. Use about
    100 ml of silver nitrate and change twice during
    impregnation. Use a chemically clean brown glass
    jar.
3. Rinse in distilled water.
4. Reduce for 1 to 2 hours in Cajal's developer.
5. Wash for 5 minutes in running tap water.
6. Dehydrate in ascending grades of alcohol. (Penfield
    points out that the time in absolute alcohol should
    be short.)
7. Clear in xylene and embed in paraffin.
8. Cut sections at 6 to 7 microns, mount on slides,
    and dry in oven as usual.
9. Hydrate sections to distilled water.
10. Tone in gold chloride solution for 5 to 10 minutes.
11. Wash in water.
12. Dehydrate in 95% alcohol, then in absolute alcohol,
    two changes, 1 minute each.
13. Clear in xylene, two changes.
14. Mount in Permount.

Note.   Sections may be counterstained in 1% safranin-0
           after gold toning. All glassware should be
           acid cleaned and glass stoppered to aviod
           precipitates.

Results.   Golgi apparatus: black. Ground substance;
           Yellow to light yellow, gray after toning.

Ref.   Da Fano, C., J. Physiol. 5, (1920), xcii-xciv

CAJAL'S SILVER-PYRIDINE METHOD FOR MEDULATED AND NONMED-
ULATED NERVE FIBERS

Fixation. 10% formalin for 12 to 24 hours.

SOLUTIONS

1.   Silver solution.

    2% aqueous silver nitrate   10 ml
    Pyridine   8 drops

2.   95% alcohol.

3.   Reducing solution.

    Hydroquinone   0.3 gm
    Distilled water   70 ml
    40% formaldehyde   30 ml

4.   Toning solution.

    1:500 aqueous yellow gold chloride.

5.   Sodium thiosulfate.

    Sodium thisosulfate   5 gm
    Distilled water   100 ml

6.   Carbol-creosote-xylene.

    Carbolic acid   10 ml
    Beechwood creosote   10 ml
    Xylene   80 ml

PROCEDURE

1.   Cut frozen sections at 30 to 40 microns into dis-
     tilled water.
2.   Wash in two changes of distilled water.
3.   Impregnate is silver pyridine solution. Leave in
     solution 5 minutes or longer at room temperature.
     Then heat over an alcohol flame to about 50°C, no
     warmer, until the sections are a clear brown color.
     Keep dish covered.
4.   Wash sections while still warm in 95% alcohol.
5.   Reduce in hydroquinone solution for 1 minute.
6.   Rinse in distilled water.
7.   Tone in yellow gold choloride for 10 minutes.
8.   Wash in distilled water.
9.   Fix in sodium thiosulfate for 10 minutes.
10. Wash in distilled water.
11. Mount sections on slide and blot with fine filter
     paper.
12. Dehydrate with 95% alcohol from a dropper bottle,
     then with absolute alcohol in the same manner.
13. Clear in carbol-creosote-xylene from a dropper bottle.

14.   Rinse in pure xylene.
15.   Mount in Permount.

Results.   Nerve fibers: deep black; if gold toning is
           used, the background has a bluish cast.   Human
           Perkinje cells are well demonstrated.

Ref.   Bolles, Lee, The Microtomist's Vade Mecum, 10
           ed., The Blakiston Co., 1946.   Used with per-
           mission of McGraw-Hill Book Co., N.Y..
           Publishers of Blakiston Volumes

BIELSCHOWSKI'S METHOD TO DEMONSTRATE NEUROFIBRILS IN
FROZEN SECTIONS

Fixation.   Tissue blocks about 3 mm-thick are fixed in
            10% formalin for 14 days.

SOLUTIONS

1.   Silver nitrate solution
     Silver nitrate   3 gm
     Distilled water   100 ml

2.   Ammoniacal silver nitrate.
     10% aqueous silver nitrate   10 ml
     40% aqueous sodium hydroxide   6 drops

     To 10 ml of silver nitrate add 6 drops of freshly
     prepared 40% sodium hydroxide, shaking between each
     drop.   The dark brown precipitate that forms should
     be then dissolved by adding 28% ammonium hydroxide,
     drop by drop, shaking between each drop and taking
     care to avoid excess ammonia.   When the precipitate
     is dissolved, bring the volume up to 25 ml with
     distilled·water.   Filter.

3.   Reducer.

     40% formaldehyde   10 ml
     Distilled water   90 ml

4.   Toning solution.

     1:500 aqueous yellow gold chloride.

5.   Sodium thiosulfate solution.

     Sodium thiosulfate   5 gm
     Distilled water   100 ml

6.   Carbol-creosote-xylene.

Carbolic acid	10 ml
Beachwood creosote	10 ml
Xylene	80 ml

PROCEDURE

1. Wash tissue blocks in running tap water for 1 hour.
2. Wash in several changes of distilled water for 24 h hours.
3. Cut frozen sections at 10 microns into distilled water.
4. Transfer sections to 3% silver nitrate for 24 hours; leave in the dark.
5. Wash in distilled water for 2 to 3 minutes.
6. Transfer sections to ammonical silver nitrate in a covered Stender dish until they take on a brown color, approximately 10 minutes. Do not allow sections to fold or overlap.
7. Rinse quickly in two changes of distilled water.
8. Reduce in 10% formalin; sections should turn uniformly black.
9. Wash in two changes of distilled water.
10. Tone in yellow gold chloride for 10 minutes.
11. Wash in distilled water.
12. Place in sodium thiosulfate for 10 minutes.
13. Wash in distilled water.
14. Mount sections on slide and blot with fine filter paper.
15. Dehydrate with 95% alcohol from a dropper bottle, then with absolute alcohol in the same manner.
16. Clear sections in carbol-creosote-xylene from a dropper bottle.
17. Rinse with pure xylene.
18. Mount in Permount.

Results. If successful, the preparation should show intracellular neurofibrils as well as axis cylinders. These are seen as black threads on a light purplish background. Reticulin fibers are impregnated to a variable degree; caution should be exerted in the interpretation.

Ref.   Mallory, F.B. Pathological Technique
         Hafner Publishing Co. New York 1968

RANSON'S PYRIDINE-SILVER METHOD TO DEMONSTRATE
NONMYELINATED FIBERS

Fixation.Absolute alcohol to which 1% of 28% ammonium
         hydroxide has been added.

SOLUTIONS

1.   Pyridine.

2.   Silver nitrate solution.

     Silver nitrate   2 gm
     Distilled water   100 ml

3.   Reducing solution.

     Pyrogallic acid   4 gm
     5% aqueous formalin   100 ml

PROCEDURE

1.   Wash tissue in distilled water for 1 to 2 minutes.
2.   Place in pyridine for 24 hours.
3.   Wash in many changes of distilled water for 24 hours.
4.   Impregnate in silver nitrate solution for 3 days in
     the dark at 35°C.
5.   Wash well in distilled water.
6.   Reduce in the pyrogallol solution for 24 to 48 hours.
7.   Rinse well in distilled water.
8.   Embed in paraffin.
9.   Cut sections at 8 microns and mount on albuminized
     slides. Dry in oven as usual.
10. Deparaffinize sections in two or three changes of
     xylene.
11. Mount in Permount.

Results. Nonmyelinated fiber: black. Myelinated fibers:
         yellow.

Ref.   Ranson, W. W., Amer. J. Anat., 12 (1911), 67-68

McMANUS' CHLORAL HYDRATE METHOD TO DEMONSTRATE NERVE
FIBERS

Fixation.10% formalin or formol-saline.

SOLUTIONS

1.   Cajal's chloral hydrate silver solution.

      Chloral hydrate   1 gm
      Silver nitrate   20 gm
      Distilled water   100 ml

2.   Bodian's hydroquinone reducer.

      Hydroquinone   1 gm
      Sodium sulfite   5 gm
      Distilled water   100 ml

      Make up fresh each time.

3.   Gold chloride toning solution.

      1% aqueous yellow gold chloride 100 ml
      Glacial acetic acid   4 drops

4.   Oxalic acid solution.

      Oxalic acid   2 gm
      Distilled water   100 ml

5.   Sodium thiosulfate solution.

      Sodium thiosulfate   5 gm
      Distilled water   100 ml

PROCEDURE

 1.   Cut paraffin section at 6 microns.
 2.   Deparaffinize and hydrate sections.
 3.   Place sections in chloral hydrate solution at 58°C
       for 30 to 60 minutes.
 4.   Wash in several changes of distilled water.
 5.   Place in Bodian's reducing solution for 10 minutes.
 6.   Wash well in distilled water.
 7.   Tone in yellow gold chloride for 10 minutes.
 8.   Wash in distilled water.
 9.   Place sections in oxalic acid until sufficiently
       reduced; fibers stand out under the microscope,
       and sections take on a gunmetal color when seen
       against a white background.
10.   Wash in distilled water, then in tap water.
11.   Place in sodium thiosulfate for 5 to 10 minutes.
12.   Wash in tap water.
13.   Dehydrate in 95% alcohol, then in absolute alcohol.
14.   Clear in xylene.

15.   Mount in Permount.

Results. Nerve fibers in human spinal cord and medulla:
          black to gray.

Ref.   McManus, J.F.A., J. Path Bact., 55 (1943), 303

BODIAN'S METHOD FOR NERVE FIBERS IN PARAFFIN SECTIONS

Fixation. 10% formalin, alcohol formalin. For nerve fibers
          in human skin, Bodian's No. 2 fixative gives
          superior results.

          Bodian's No. 2 fixative

          40% formaldehyde   5 ml
          Glacial acetic acid   5 ml
          80% alcohol   90 ml

SOLUTIONS

1.   Protargol solution.*

      Protargol   1 gm
      Distilled water   100 ml

      Dust the Protargol carefully and slowly over the
      surface of the distilled water in a wide dish; do
      not agitate, - allow to dissolve slowly. Add 4 to 6
      gm of metallic copper shot,† per 100 ml of Protargol
      to staining dish before placing sections in solution.
      (Copper shot should be cleaned in nitric acid and
      washed in distilled water before use.)

2.   Reducing solution. (Make up fresh each time.)

      Hydroquimone   1 gm
      Sodium sulfite   5 gm
      Distilled water   100 ml

3.   Toning solution.

      1% yellow gold chloride containing 3 drops of
      glacial acetic acid per 100 ml of solution.

*Protargol, Roboz Surgical Instrument Co., Washington,
 D. C.
†Copper shot, Merck and Co. After use, copper shot can
 be cleaned in nitric acid, washed well in running tap
 water, dried, and reused.

4.   Oxalic acid solution.

      Oxalic acid   2 gm
      Distilled water   100 ml

5.   Sodium thiosulfate solution.

      Sodium thiosulfate   5 gm
      Distilled water   100 ml

PROCEDURE

1.   Cut paraffin sections at 10 to 15 microns.
2.   Deparaffinize and hydrate sections to distilled
      water.
3.   Place in Protargol solution in closed staining dish
      for 24 to 48 hours at 37°C.
4.   Rinse in distilled water. (Transfer sections to
      clean Coplin jar.)
5.   Reduce in hydroquinone solution for 10 minutes.
6.   Wash well in distilled water.
7.   Tone in gold chloride for 10 minutes.
8.   If sections do not have a light purple color, place
      in oxalic acid solution for 5 minutes.
9.   Wash in tap water for 5 minutes.
10.   Fix in sodium thiosulfate for 5 minutes.
11.   Wash in tap water.
12.   Dehydrate in 95% alcohol then absolute alcohol.
13.   Clear in xylene.
14.   Mount in Permont.

Results. Myelinated fibers, nonmyelinated fibers, the
         endfeet of Held and neurofibrils: black.

Ref.   Bodian, D. A., Anat. Record, 65 (1936), 89-97.

PENFIELD'S SECOND MODIFICATION FOR OLIGODENDROGLIA AND
MICROGLIA

Fixation. Formalin-ammonium-bromide; 10% formalin for
          about 1 week gives excellent results.

SOLUTIONS

1.   Globus hydrobromic acid.

      Hydrobromic acid 40%   5 ml
      Distilled water   95 ml

2.   Mordant solution.

      Sodium carbonate   5 gm
      Distilled water   100 ml

3.   Hortega's weak silver carbonate solution.

      10% aqueous silver nitrate   5 ml
      5% aqueous sodium carbonate   20 ml

      With a dropper bottle add fresh 28% ammonium
      hydroxide drop by drop until the precipiate just
      dissolved, do not add ammonia to excess. Keep
      the solution in motion while adding the ammonia.
      Filter through a Whatman No. 1 filter paper; bring
      the volume up to 75 ml with distilled water.

4.   Reducer.

      40% formaldehyde   1 ml
      Distilled water   99 ml

5.   Toning solution.

      1:500 aqueous yellow gold chloride.

6.   Fixing solution.

      Sodium thiosulfate   5 gm
      Distilled water   100 ml

7.   Carbol-creosote-xylene.

      Beechwood creosote   10 ml
      Carbolic acid (melted crystals)   10 ml
      Xylene   80 ml

PROCEDURE

1.   Cut frozen sections at 20 to 25 microns into dis-
      tilled water or 1% formalin.

2. Deformalinize sections in a Petri dish of distilled water containing 10 to 15 drops of 28%
   ammonium hydroxide. Cover the dish to prevent the
   escape of ammonia and leave overnight.
3. Bromurate in hydrobromic acid solution at 37°C for
   1 hour.
4. Wash in three changes of distilled water.
5. Mordant in sodium carbonate for 1 hour. Sections
   may be left in solution up to 5 hours without harm.
6. Impregnate with or without washing in Hortega's
   weak silver bath for 3 to 5 minutes or until they
   are a smooth gray.
7. Transfer sections at intervals of 30 seconds to reducer and examine under microsope. If it is desired to impregnate microglia, agitate the sections
   by blowing on the surface of the reducer, better
   impregnation of oligodendroglia is obtained if the
   sections are allowed to float to the bottom of the
   dish without agitation. Discard solution as it
   discolors.
8. Wash in distilled water.
9. Tone in 1:500 yellow gold chloride for 10 minutes
   or until section appears bluish gray.
10. Wash in distilled water.
11. Fix in sodium thiosulfate for 5 minutes.
12. Wash well in distilled water.
13. Mount sections on slide and blot with fine filter
    paper; dehydrate with absolute alcohol from a
    dropper bottle.
14. Clear with carbol-creosote-xylene.
15. Rinse with pure xylene.
16. Mount in Permount.

Results. By this method both oligodendroglai and micro-
         glia can be demonstrated with a considerable
         degree of consistency. There may be a faint
         staining of astrocytes if the sections are
         left too long in silver.

         McCarter's modification. At step 5 mordant in
         in the following solution for 1 hours, (but the
         sections may remain indefinitely).

         Sodium carbonate 5% aqueous   15 ml
         Aliumium and ammonium sulfate 5% aqueous   15 ml

         This modification enhances the staining of
         oligodendroglia processes against a clearer
         background.

Ref.   Penfield, W. G., Amer. J. Path. 4 (1928), 153-157
            McCarter, J. C., Amer. J. Path. 16 (1940) 233-236
            Globus, J. H., Arch, Neurol. Psychiat., 18
            (1927), 263-271

DEL RIO-HORTEGA'S SILVER CARBONATE METHOD FOR OLIGODENDROGLIA

Fixation. Formalin-ammonium-bromide for at least 24 hours,
        hours, not exceeding 48 hours.

SOLUTIONS

1.   Hortega's silver carbonate solution.

       10% aqueous silver nitrate   5 ml
       5% aqueous sodium carbonate   20 ml

       With a dropper bottle add fresh 28% ammonium
       hydroxide drop by drop until the precipitate is
       just dissolved, do not add ammonia to excess. Keep
       the solution in motion while adding the ammonia.
       Filter through a Whatman No. 1 filter paper, and
       bring the volume up to 45 ml with distilled water
       (strong solution). Hortega's weak silver carbonate
       solution: bring the volume up to 75 ml with dis-
       tilled water; undiluted, add no water.

2.   Putt's modification.

       10% aqueous silver nitrate   40 ml
       5% aqueous sodium carbonate   80 ml

       Dissolve the precipitate with 28% ammonium hydroxide
       as above; filter but do not add distilled water.

3.   Reducer.

       40% formaldehyde   1 ml
       Distilled water   99 ml

4.   Toning solution.

       1:500 aqueous yellow gold chloride.

5.   Fixing solution.

       Sodium thiosulfate   5 gm
       Distilled water   100 ml

6.   Carbol-creosote-xylene.

Beechwood creosote	10 ml
Carbolic acid	10 ml
Xylene	80 ml

PROCEDURE

1.   Cut frozen sections at 20 to 25 microns into dis-
     tilled water. If the sections are left in water
     for more than a few hours, the oligodendroglia will
     swell. This can be avoided by adding a few drops
     of 40% formalin to the water.
2.   Transfer sections through three changes of distilled
     water in Petri dishes, adding 10 to 15 drops of 28%
     ammonium hydroxide to the first dish. Rinse for 1
     to 2 minutes in each change.
3.   Impregnate sections in silver carbonate solution
     at room temperature for 1 to 5 minutes. Sections
     should be transfered to the reducer at intervals of
     about 30 seconds. At times, depending on the tis-
     sue, the silver carbonate solution should be varied
     by using Hortega's strong solution or Putt's
     undiluted solution. This can be determined after
     reduction.
4.   Reduce a section in 1% formalin until grayish
     black; usually if the section takes on a gray met-
     allic dross, the impregnation is successful, - a
     transparent walnut color indicates poor demonstration
     of expansions. Microglia can better be demonstrated
     by blowing on the surface of the silver bath, keep-
     ing the section in constant agitation. For oligo-
     dendroglia, allow the section to settle gently on
     the bottom of the bath. Discard solution as it
     discolors.
5.   Wash in distilled water. At this point the section
     may be examined under the microscope. When the
     desired staining time is achieved, a number of
     sections can be carried through the silver bath and
     reducer.
6.   Tone in 1/500 yellow gold chloride for 10 minutes
     or until the sections are bluish gray.
7.   Wash in distilled water.
8.   Fix in thiosulfate solution for 5 minutes.
9.   Wash in distilled water.
10. Mount sections on slide and blot with fine filter
     paper, dehydrate with absolute alcohol from a
     dropper bottle.
11. Clear in carbol-creosote-xylene from dropper bottle.

12.   Rinse in pure xylene.
13.   Mount in Permount.

Results. Oligodendroglia and microglia are impregnated
          a gray or grayish black against a lighter back-
          ground. Astrocytes and the bodies of neurons
          are less fully demonstrated.

Note.   This is a capricious method mostly due to pro-
          longed fixation which sometimes can be corrected
          by varying the silver baths from strong to weak
          or Putt's modification.

Ref.   Hortega, Del Rio P., Bol. Real Soc. Esp. Hist.
          Nat., 1921.

DEL RIO-HORTEGA'S LITHIUM SILVER CARBONATE METHOD FOR
ASTROCYTES

Fixation. Formalin-ammonium-bromide for 3 weeks, 10%
           formalin (see step 2).

SOLUTIONS

1.   Globus hydrobromic acid solution.

      Hydrobromic acid 40%   5 ml
      Distilled water   95 ml

2.   Lithium silver carbonate.

      Saturated aqueous lithium carbonate   20 ml
      10% aqueous silver nitrate   5 ml

      With a dropper bottle add, drop by drop, enough
      fresh 28% ammonium hydroxide to dissolve the
      precipitate. Agitate gently; do not add ammonia to
      excess. Make up to 75 ml with distilled water and
      filter through a Whatman No. 1 filter paper.

3.   Reducer.

      40% formaldehyde   1 ml
      Distilled water.   99 ml

4.   Toning solution.

      1:500 aqueous yellow gold chloride

5.   Fixing solution.

Sodium thiosulfate   5 gm
Distilled water   100 ml

6.   Carbol-creosote-xylene.

Beechwood creosote   10 ml
Carbolic acid   100 ml
Xylene   80 ml

PROCEDURE

1. Cut frozen sections at 15 to 20 microns into dis-
    tilled water in a Petri dish containing 10 to 15
    drops of 40% formaldehyde.
2. Bromurate formalin-fixed material in hydrobromic
    acid for 1 hour at 37°C.
3. Wash well in three changes of distilled water, the
    first containing 2 to 3 drops of 28% ammonium
    hydroxide.
4. Impregnate 6 to 7 sections in a Stender dish con-
    taining the lithium silver solution plus a few
    drops of pyriding to prevent the formation of scum
    on the surface. Cover with a watch glass and place
    over an alcohol flame, heat to 45 -50°C, gently
    agitating the dish from time to time. Leave sec-
    tions in solution until they develop an amber color,
    usually 3 to 5 minutes. At times the addition of
    10 to 12 drops of 95% alcohol improves the im-
    pregnation.
5. Wash sections in distilled water, allow the sections
    to fall to the bottom of the dish, 3 to 4 seconds.
    Prolonged washing is detrimental.
6. Reduce in 1% formalin for a few seconds.
7. Wash well in distilled water.
8. Tone in 1:500 gold chloride for 5 to 10 minutes.
    Sections will take on a gray color, heat solution
    not exceeding 50°C, until sections turn purple.
9. Wash well in distilled water.
10. Fix in sodium thiosulfate for 5 minutes.
11. Mount sections on slides and blot with fine filter
    paper, dehydrate wtih absolute alcohol from a
    dropper bottle.
12. Clear sections with carbol-creosote-xylene mixture
    from dropper bottle.
13. Rinse in xylene.
14. Mount in Permount.

Results.   Astrocytes and their processes: blackish on a
              purple background. Oligodendroglia and micro-
              glia: not impregnated. The bodies of neurons,
              axis cylinders, and reticulin fibers and fre-
              quently demonstrated.

Ref.   Hortega, Del Rio P., Trab Lab. Invest. Biol.
              Univ. Madrid, 15 (1917), 367

HORTEGA'S SILVER CARBONATE METHOD FOR MICROGLIA

Fixation.   Cajal's formalin-ammonium-bromide for 12 to
              48 hours. Place in fresh solution for 10 min-
              utes in oven at 50°C before sectioning.

SOLUTIONS

1.   Hortega's weak silver carbonate solution.

      10% aqueous silver nitrate   5 ml
      5% aqueous sodium carbonate   10 ml

      With a dropper bottle add fresh 28% ammonium hydrox-
      ide drop by drop until the precipitate is just dis-
      solved; do not add ammonia to excess. Filter
      through a Whatman No. 1 filter paper. Bring the
      volume up to 75 ml with distilled water.

2.   Reducer.

      40% formaldehyde   1 ml
      Distilled water   99 ml

3.   Toning solution.

      1:500 yellow gold chloride

4.   Fixing solution.

      Sodium thiosulfate   5 gm
      Distilled water   100 ml

5.   Carbol-creosote-xylene.

      Beechwood creosote   10 ml
      Carbolic acid   10 ml
      Xylene   80 ml

PROCEDURE

1. Cut frozen sections at 20 to 25 microns into dis-
    tilled water.
2. Transfer to three changes of distilled water in
    Petri dishes, adding 10 to 15 drops of 28% ammonium
    hydroxide to the first dish. Rinse for 1 to 2 min-
    utes in each change.
3. Impregnate sections in silver carbonate solution at
    room temperature for up to 2 minutes. Remove sec-
    tions at intervals of 20 seconds and transfer to
    reducer.
4. Reduce with gentle agitation with glass "hockey
    stick" until sections take on a uniform grayish color.
    Discard solution as it darkens.
5. Wash in distilled water.
6. Tone in 1:500 yellow gold chloride for 10 minutes.
7. Wash in distilled water.
8. Fix in thiosulfate solution for 5 minutes.
9. Wash in distilled water.
10. Mount on slides and blot with fine filter paper;
    dehydrate with absolute alcohol from dropper bottle.
11. Clear with carbol-creosote-xylene from dropper
    bottle.
12. Rinse in pure xylene.
13. Mount in Permount.

Results.   Microglia and expansions: black against a
            lighter background.

Note.   Rinse glass hockey stick in distilled water
            between solution changes. Lipids may be dem-
            onstrated in microglia by staining in Putt's
            flaming red lipid stain after step 9. The
            sections must then be mounted in Kaiser's
            glycerin jelly.

Ref.   Hortega, Del Rio Pa., Arch. Cardoil. Haematol.,
            2 (1921b), 161.

CAJAL'S GOLD CHLORIDE-SUBLIMATE METHOD TO DEMONSTRATE
ASTROCYTES

Fixation.   The optimum fixation is obtained after 24
            hours in formalin-ammonium bromide. Proto-
            plasmic astrocytes can best be demonstrated
            after a short period of fixation, fibrous
            astrocytes after a longer one.

SOLUTIONS

1.   Cajal's gold chloride solution.

         Mercuric chloride, crystalline, not
         powdered.   0.5 gm
         Distilled water   50 ml
         1% aqueous brown gold chloride (Merck)   10 ml

         Dissolve the mercuric chloride in the distilled
         water with the aid of gentle heat over a small flame.
         Do not overheat; cool and filter. Prepare fresh
         each time.

         Putt's modification: Increase the mercuric chloride
         to 1 gm.

2.   Sodium thiosulfate (hypo).

         Sodium thiosulfate   5 gm
         Distilled water   100 ml

3.   Carbol-creosote-xylene.

         Beechwood creosote   10 ml
         Carbolic acid   10 ml
         Xylene   80 ml

PROCEDURE

1.   Cut frozen sections at 20 to 25 microns into distill-
     ed water in a Petri dish containing 10 to 15 drops
     of 40% formaldehyde.
2.   Rinse well in 2 to 3 changes of distilled water.
3.   Impregnate sections in the gold bath in a covered
     Petri dish for 3 hours or more at room temperature.
     Place dish on a white background to observe impreg-
     nation. Do not allow sections to overlap in the
     gold bath. They should rest on the bottom of the
     dish. Sections may be rinsed in distilled water,
     mounted wet on a slide and examined under the micro-
     scope to check staining. It is not necessary to
     carry out this procedure in the dark.
4.   Wash well in distilled water.
5.   Fix in sodium thiosulfate solution until sections
     become flexible, 5 minutes.
6.   Wash in distilled water.
7.   Mount sections on slides and blot with fine filter
     paper. Dehydrate with absolute alcohol from dropper
     bottle.

8. Clear sections with carbol-creosote-xylene from dropper bottle.
9. Wash well with pure xylene from a dropper bottle.
10. Mount in Permount.

Results.   The astrocytes with their processes appear as spider-shaped cells, varying in tint from deep ruby to purplish black, according to the length of time in the gold bath against a light ruby background. The nuclei of other cells are faintly seen, while capillaries are more strongly defined. The method is not consistent in its staining of tumor cells in gliomas.

Note.   Favorable staining of astrocytes by the gold method may be carried out on fresh formalin fixed material; however the results are inferior to formalin-ammonium-bromide fixation which seems to lessen the tendency to granular staining. Sometimes formalin-fixed tissue may be refixed in formalin-ammonium-bromide with improved results.

            If tissue is left for an extended period in formalin or formalin-ammonium-bromide all astrocytes (protoplasmic and fibrous) become refractory to the gold stain.

            The gold chloride solution keeps well in a glass stoppered brown bottle.

Ref.   Cajal, Ramon y, Trab. Lab. Invest. Biol. Madrid, 11 (1913), 219; 14 (1916), 155.

DEL RIO-HORTEGA'S MODIFICATION OF CAJAL'S GOLD CHLORIDE-SUBLIMATE METHOD FOR ASTROCYTES

Fixation.   Tissues may be fixed up to 30 days in formalin-ammonium-bromide.

SOLUTIONS

1. Hortega's modified gold solution.

    1:500 aqueous yellow gold chloride   50 ml
    Mercuric chloride, crystalline, not
    powdered.   1 gm
    Glacial acetic acid   20 drops

Dissolve the mercuric chloride in the yellow gold
solution with the aid of gentle heat. Filter and
add the glacial acetic acid. Prepare fresh each
time.

2.   Oxalic acid solution.

Oxalic acid	5	gm
Distilled water	100	ml

3.   Sodium thiosulfate   5 gm
      Distilled water   100 ml

4.   Carbol-creosote-xylene.

Beechwood creosote	10	ml
Carbolic acid	10	ml
Xylene	80	ml

PROCEDURE

1.   Cut frozen sections at 20 to 25 microns into dis-
      tilled water.
2.   Wash sections in distilled water in a Petri dish con-
      taining a few drops of 28% ammonium hydroxide for 2
      to 3 minutes.
3.   Impregnate sections in gold solution in a covered
      Petri dish at 30 to 35°C until they are a deep ruby
      color. Do not allow sections to overlap. Sections
      should rest on the bottom of the dish.
4.   Rinse in distilled water. Examine under microscope.
5.   If stain does not appear intense enough, place in
      oxalic acid solution for 5 to 10 minutes.
6.   Wash in distilled water.
7.   Fix in sodium thiosulfate solution containing a few
      drops of 28% ammonium hydroxide for 5 minutes.
8.   Wash in distilled water.
9.   Mount on a slide, blot with fine filter paper, and
      dehydrate with absolute alcohol from a dropper bottle.
10.   Clear sections with carbol-creosote-xylene from a
      dropper bottle.
11.   Rinse in pure xylene.
12.   Mount in Permount.

Results.   The astrocytes and their processes appear as
            spider-shaped cells.

Note.   This method was devised by Hortega for the
               staining of immature glia cells in the gliomas
               because Cajal's method does not give consist-
               ently good results. The method works well for
               normal material, especially man, cat, and dog,
               but not well in rabbit.

Ref.   Prados, M., personal communication.

HOLZER'S METHOD TO DEMONSTRATE GLIA FIBERS

Fixation.   10% formalin.

SOLUTIONS

1.   0.5% aqueous phosphomolybdic acid, fresh
       solution   10 ml
       95% alcohol   20 ml

2.   Alcohol-chloroform mixture

       Absolute alcohol   20 ml
       Chloroform   80 ml

3.   Crystal violet stain.

       Crystal violet   5 gm
       Absolute alcohol   20 ml
       Chloroform   80 ml

4.   Potassium bromide solution.

       Potassium bromide   10 gm
       Distilled water   100 ml

5.   Differentiating solution.

       Aniline oil   40 ml
       Chloroform   60 ml
       1% aqueous acetic acid   10 drops

PROCEDURE

1.   Cut frozen sections at 20 microns into distilled
     water or water with a few drops of 40% formaldehyde.
2.   Place sections in 50% alcohol for 30 minutes to 2
     hours.
3.   Mount sections carefully on slide and blot carefully
     with filter paper. Or embed tissue in paraffin and

cut sections at 8 to 10 microns, deparaffinize and hydrate sections to distilled water.

4. Carry sections individually through the following solutions.
5. Place in phosphomolybdic acid solution for 3 minutes.
6. Blot section with filter paper that has been moistened with the absolute alcohol-chloroform mixture.
7. Pour the absolute alcohol-chloroform mixture over the section from a dropper bottle until it appears a homogeneous gray.
8. Drain off the excess absolute alcohol-chloroform mixture, place slide on a staining rack, pour on the crystal violet solution from a pipette, and stain for 30 seconds. Drain.
9. Blot sections well with filter paper.
10. From a dropper bottle pour on the potassium bromide solution and wash well until waves of color disappear.
11. Differentiate in the aniline-chloroform-acetic acid solution for 30 seconds; control under microscope.
12. Clear in two or three changes of xylene.
13. Mount in Permount.

Results.   Glia fibers: blue. Background: violet.

Note.   Prepare all solutions in advance, from the time in phosphomolybdic acid, staining should be completed in no more than 5 minutes. All glassware should be clean and dry.

Ref.   Carleton's Histological Technique Drury, R. A. B. Wallington, E. A. (ed), Oxford University Press, 4th ed, 1967, London.

MALLORY'S ANILINE BLUE ORANGE-G METHOD FOR NEUROGLIA FIBERS AND CELLS

Fixation.   Helly's or Zenker's fluids preferred; 10% formalin may be used.

SOLUTIONS

1. Mordant solution.

    Iron alum (ferric ammonium sulfate)   1 gm
    Sulfuric acid   1 ml
    50% alcohol   98 ml

2. Fuchsin solution.

Acid fuchsin	0.5 gm
Glacial acetic acid	7 drops
Distilled water	100 ml

3. Aniline blue solution.

Aniline blue (water soluble)	0.5 gm
Orange-G	2 gm
Oxalic acid	2 gm
Distilled water	100 ml

PROCEDURE

1. Deparaffinize and hydrate sections.
2. Remove mercury crystals if necessary.
3. Place in mordant solution for 10 to 30 minutes.
4. Wash well in distilled water.
5. Stain in acid fuchsin solution for 1 to 2 minutes.
6. Wash well in distilled water.
7. Stain in aniline blue solution for 15 minutes.
8. Differentiate in absolute alcohol, two changes.
9. Clear in xylene, two changes.
10. Mount in Permount.

Results.   Glia fibers: violet. Glia cells and axis
            cylinders: blue. Myelin: gold with a slight
            rose tint. Ganglion cells and nessel walls:
            dark blue. Nucleoli and blood corpuscles:
            bright red. Nuclei: greenish yellow.

Ref.   Mallory, F. B., Patholigical Technique, Hafner
            Publishing Co., New York, 1961.

KLÜVER'S AND BARRERA'S LUXOL FAST BLUE METHOD TO DEMONSTRATE
MYELIN

Fixation. 10% formalin.

SOLUTIONS

1. Luxol fast blue solution.

Luxol fast blue MBSN* (solvent blue 38)	1 gm

*Luxol fast blue MBSN, E. I. du Pont de Nemours & Co.,
Organic Chemical Department Wilmington, Del.

95% alcohol   1000 ml
Glacial acetic acid 10% aqueous   5 ml

Filter before using. Solution stable for one year.

2. Lithium carbonate solution.

Lithium carbonate 1% aqueous   5 ml
Distilled water   95 ml

3. Cresyl fast violet (echt).*

Cresyl fast violet   0.1 gm
Distilled water   100 ml

Add 5 drops of 10% glacial acetic acid to every 30
ml of solution just before use; filter.

4. 70% alcohol

Absolute alcohol   70 ml
Distilled water   30 ml

PROCEDURE

1. Cut paraffin sections at 15 microns.
2. Deparaffinize sections in 95% alcohol, several
   changes.
3. Place sections in luxol fast blue solution overnight
   in 60°C oven in a well covered staining jar.
4. Immerse in 95% alcohol to remove excess stain.
5. Wash in distilled water.
6. Rinse sections for 2 to 3 seconds in lithium carbonate
   solution to begin differentiation.
7. Continue differentiation in 70% alcohol until gray
   and white matter can be distinguished; do not overdifferentiate.
8. Wash in distilled water.
9. Rinse sections in lithium carbonate solution for 3
   to 5 seconds, no longer.
10. Complete differentiation in 70% alcohol until the
    white matter is stained a greenish - blue in contrast
    with the colorless gray matter.
11. Wash thoroughly in distilled water.
12. Stain for 6 minutes in warm, freshly filtered cresyl
    violet solution.
13. Rinse in distilled water.

*Cresyl fast violet, C. I. No. 51010, Roboz Surgical
Instrument Co., Washington, D. C.

14. Differentiate in several changes of 95% alcohol until the alcohol is no longer tinted.
15. Dehydrate in absolute alcohol.
16. Clear in xylene.
17. Mount in Permount.

Results.   Myelinated fibers: greenish blue. Nissl cells: reddish.

Note.   T. N. Salthouse, recommends Luxol Fast Blue ARN (solvent blue 37), Stain Tech., 37 (1962) 313-316.

Ref.   Kluver, H. and Barrera, E., J. Neuropath. Exper. Neurol., 12 (1953), 400-403.

MARGOLIS' AND PICKETT'S LUXOL FAST BLUE-PAS-HEMATOXYLIN METHOD

Fixation. 10% formalin.

SOLUTIONS

1. Luxol fast blue solution.

   Luxol fast blue MBSN* (solvent blue   0.1 gm
   38)
   95% alcohol   100 ml

   Dissolve the dye in the alcohol. Add 5 ml of 10% aqueous glacial acetic acid to every 1000 ml. This solution keeps indefinitely.

2. Lithium carbonate solution.

   Lithium carbonate   0.05 gm
   Distilled water   100 ml

3. Periodic acid solution.

   Periodic acid   0.5 gm
   Distilled water   100 ml

4. Normal hydrochloric acid.

   Hydrochloric acid, sp. gr. 1.19   83.5 ml
   Distilled water   916.5 ml

*Luxol fast blue MBSN, E. I. du Pont de Nemours & Co. Organic Chemical Department Wilmington Del.

5. Schiff's reagent. Bring 200 ml of distilled water
    to a boil, remove from flame, add 1 gm of basic
    fuchsin, and stir until dissolved. Cool to 50°C.
    Filter and add 20 ml of normal hydrochloric acid.
    Cool further to 25°C. Add 1 gm of sodium or potassium
    metabisulfite. (Na2S205, K2S205). Place in the dark
    in a stoppered bottle for 18 to 24 hours; solution
    takes on an orange color. Add 0.5 gm of activated
    charcoal and shake well, then filter through a coarse
    filter paper. Store under refrigeration in a brown
    stoppered bottle of the same volume. Solution is
    stable for several weeks. Use at room temperature.

6. Sulfurous acid rinse.

10% aqueous sodium metabisulfite	6 ml
Normal hydrochloric acid	5 ml
Distilled water	100 ml

7. Papamiltiades' hematoxylin.

Hematoxylin; 1% aqueous solution	100 ml
Aluminum sulfate: 5% aqueous solution	50 ml
Zinc sulfate: 4% aqueous solution	25 ml
Potassium iodide: 4% aqueous solution	25 ml
Glacial acetic acid	8 ml
Glycerin	25 ml

    Can be used immediately; effective for about 2 months.

PROCEDURE

1. Deparaffinize sections to 95% alcohol, several changes.
2. Place sections in luxol fast blue overnight in 60°C
    oven.
3. Rinse off excess stain in 95% alcohol.
4. Rinse in distilled water.
5. Place in lithium carbonate solution for a few seconds.
6. Differentiate in 70% alcohol for 20 to 30 seconds.
7. Rinse in distilled water.
8. Place in a fresh solution of lithium carbonate for
    20 to 30 seconds.
9. Complete differentiation in 70% alcohol until the
    white matter is stained a greenish - blue in sharp
    contrast with the colorless gray matter.
10. Rinse in distilled water.
11. Place in periodic acid solution for 5 minutes.
12. Rinse in two changes of distilled water.
13. Place in Schiff's solution for 15 to 30 minutes.
14. Rinse in sulfurous acid solution, three changes
    of 2 minutes each.

15. Wash in tap water for 5 minutes.
16. Stain in Papamiltiade's hematoxylin for 1 minute.
17. Wash in tap water for 5 minutes.
18. If background in not clear, differentiate for 1 second in acid alcohol and wash well. If nuclei are not dark enough, blue in weak ammonia water; wash well.
19. Dehydrate in 95% alcohol, then in absolute alcohol two changes, 1 to 2 minutes each.
20. Clear in xylene.
21. Mount in Permount.

Results. Myelin sheaths, erythrocytes: blue-green. Nuclei: blue-black. Capillary walls: red. PAS positive elements: rose to red.

Ref. Margolis, G. and Pickett, J. P., Lab. Invest., 5 (1956) Copyright The Williams and Wilkins Co. 459-474. Papamiltiades, M.: Acta Anatomic, 19, 1953.

SWANK-DAVENPORT OSMIUM TETROXIDE-FORMALIN METHOD FOR DEGENERATING MYELIN

Fixation. Tissue blocks 3 mm thick are placed in 10% formalin without perfusion.

SOLUTIONS

1.	1% aqueous potassium chlorate	60 ml
	1% aqueous osmium tetroxide	20 ml
	Glacial acetic acid	1 ml
	40% formaldehyde	12 ml

PROCEDURE

1. Place tissue blocks directly into the osmium tetroxide solution for 7 to 10 days. - Approximately 15 volumes of solution to 1 volume of tissue. During staining, the solution should be agitated daily and the pieces of tissue turned over. A chemically clean brown glass stoppered bottle should be used.
2. Wash tissue for 24 hours in running tap water.
3. Embed tissue in celloidin or in paraffin.
4. Paraffin sections should be dehydrated in acetone and cleared in petroleum ether and infiltrated with paraffin in the vacuum oven.
5. Cut celloidin sections at 15 microns, paraffin at 6 microns.

6. Deparaffinize in chloroform and mount in Permount.
7. Dehydrate celloidin sections in 70% alcohol, then
    in equal parts of ethyl alcohol and butyl alcohol,
    and finally in pure butyl alcohol.
8. Clear in xylene.
9. Mount in Permount.

Results.   Foci of degeneration are stained black.

Note.   Osmium tetroxide solutions are very sensitive
           to contamination and should be made up in
           chemically clean glassware with the purest
           distilled water. The solution is good as long
           as it remains colorless. It attacks the eyes
           and throat and should be used in a well vent-
           ilated room or under a hood. Pour used
           solutions directly down the drain and flush
           with cold water.

Ref.   Swank, R. L., and Davenport, H. A., Stain
           Tech., 10 (1953) 2. Swank, R. L., and Daven-
           port, H. A., Stain Tech., 10 (1953) 3..
           Copyright The Williams and Wilkins Co.

MARCHI'S METHOD FOR FATTY DEGENERATION IN MYELIN SHEATHS

Fixation. Muller's fluid. Tissue should remain in
           Muller's fluid for 8 days to 5 weeks depending
           on the size of the blocks. The solution should
           be changed daily for the first week and once
           thereafter

SOLUTIONS

1. Muller's fluid.

    Potassium dichromate   2.5 gm
    Sodium sulfate   1 gm
    Distilled water   100 ml

2. Marchi's fluid: prepare fresh.

    Muller's fluid   100 ml
    Osmium trioxide 1% aqueous   50 ml

PROCEDURE

1. After fixation, transfer blocks of tissue directly
    to Marchi's fluid for 4 to 30 days. Keep in the
    dark. Change fluid as it blackens. Brain tissue re-
    quires 20 to 30 days, spinal cord 8 to 12 days.

2. Wash blocks for 24 hours in running tap water.
3. Dehydrate blocks fairly rapidly and embed in paraffin
    for cellular studies. Chloroform should be used in-
    stead of xylene or toluene as a clearing agent. For
    tract preparations embed in celliodin in the usual
    manner. Keep embedding steps to a minimum.
4. Section paraffin blocks at 6 microns; counterstain
    lightly with Van Gieson's picro-fuchsin if desired.
    Cut celloidin sections at 20 microns.
5. Dehydrate in 95% alcohol, then in absolute alcohol.
    Clear in chloroform and mount in chloroform-resin.
    Clear celloidin sections in oil of origanum after
    95% alcohol and mount in chloroform-resin.

Results.   Foci of degeneration: black. Neutral fats:
            black. Background: yellowish.

Ref.   Marchi, V. and Algeri, G. Riv. Sperm. Freniat.,
            11 (1885), 492-494. Mallory, F. B.,
            Pathological Technique, Hafner Publishing Co.,
            New York, 1968.

Note.   This method can be used to demonstrate fatty
            changes in the nerve cells. It is applicable
            only to medullated fibers; the effects of a
            lesion is not demonstrable until a week after
            its occurence.

SCHROEDER'S METHOD TO DEMONSTRATE MYELIN

Fixation. 10% formalin.

SOLUTIONS

1. Solution A: Muller's fluid   Solution B: Weigert's
                                  1st mordant.
    Potassium dichromate 2.5 gm   Potassium dichromate 5 gm
    Sodium sulfate   1 gm   Chromium fluoride   2.5 gm
    Distilled water   100 gm   Distilled water   100 gm
    Filter   Boil and filter

2. Working mordant solution.

    Solution A: 2 parts   Solution B: 1 part

3. Staining solution.

    10% hematoxylin in absolute alcohol   3 ml
    Distilled water   100 ml

Boil for 5 minutes, cool, and add 3 ml of saturated
lithium carbonate. Bring volume up to 100 ml with
distilled water.

4. Differentiating solution.

Potassium permanganate   0.25 gm
Distilled water   100 gm

5. Pal's solution.

Oxalic acid   1 gm
Potassium sulfate   1 gm
Distilled water   100 ml

Make up fresh solution just before use.

6. Saturated aqueous lithium carbonate   1 ml
    Distilled water   100 ml

PROCEDURE

1. Cut frozen sections at 20 to 30 microns into dis-
    tilled water.
2. Place sections in mordant solution at 37°C overnight.
    Do not allow sections to fold or overlap.
3. Rinse tissue in distilled water.
4. Stain in hematoxylin for 12 hours (overnight) at
    room temperature.
5. Wash in distilled water; sections may be left for
    several hours.
6. Differentiate in potassium permanganate for 15 seconds.
7. Rinse in distilled water.
8. Differentiate in Pal's solution for 1 minute; agitate
    sections gently.
9. Wash in distilled water and examine under microscope,
    If sections are overstained, repeat steps 6, 7, and
    8. Do not overdifferentiate.
10. Place sections in lithium carbonate solution for 1
    minute.
11. Wash in several changes of distilled water for 1 day.
12. Dehydrate in 95% alcohol, then in absolute alcohol.
13. Clear in two or three changes of xylene.
14. Mount in Permount.

Results. Myelin: blue-black against a colorless back-
          ground.

Ref.   Gray, P. The Microtonists Formulary and Guide
          Constable Publishers London England

WEIGERT-PAL METHOD TO DEMONSTRATE MYELIN SHEATHS

Fixation. Muller's fluid for 2 weeks or more or 10% formalin, followed by Muller's fluid for 2 weeks or more depending on the size of the block.

Muller's fluid

Potassium dichromate	2.5 gm
Sodium sulfate	1 gm
Distilled water	100 ml

The solution should be changed weekly during fixation.

SOLUTIONS

1. Weigert's hematoxylin.

Hematoxylin crystals	10 gm
Absolute alcohol	100 ml

Ripen for 2 to 3 months.

2. Working solution.

Ripened hematoxylin	1 ml
Distilled water	90 ml
Saturated aqueous lithium carbonate	1-2 ml

3. Differentiating solution No. 1.

Potassium permanganate	0.25 gm
Distilled water	100 ml

4. Pal's solution.

Oxalic acid	1 gm
Potassium sulfate	1 gm
Distilled water	200 ml

Make up fresh solution just before use.

5. Carbol xylene.

Xylene	300 ml
Phenol crystals	100 gm

PROCEDURE

1. Wash fixed tissue blocks in running tap water for
    6 to 12 hours.
2. Embed tissue in celloidin.
3. Cut spinal cord sections at 20 microns, cortex at
    30 microns.
4. Place sections in Weigert's hematoxylin for 24 to 48
    hours at room temperature or for 2 hours in 37°C
    oven. Sections may become brittle with heat.
5. Wash in water to which has been added 2 to 3
    drops of saturated lithium carbonate.
6. Place in potassium permanganate solution for 10
    to 15 seconds.
7. Wash in tap water.
8. Differentiate in Pal's solution, alternating with
    potassium permanganate; rinse sections in water be-
    tween solutions until only the myelinated nerve
    fiber are blue. Do not leave sections in differen-
    tiating solutions too long, especially the potassium
    permanaganate; otherwise overdifferentiation will
    result, which is irreversible.
9. Wash thoroughly in tap water.
10. Dehydrate in 95% alcohol.
11. Clear in carbol-xylene, two or three changes.
12. Clear in fresh xylene.
13. Mount in Permount.

Results. Myelin sheaths: deep black. Background:
          unstained.

Ref.   Mallory, F. B., Pathological Technique, Hafner
          Publishing Co., New York, 1968.

SPIELMEYER'S METHOD TO DEMONSTRATE MYELIN IN FROZEN
SECTIONS

Fixation. 10% formalin for at least 3 days.

SOLUTIONS

1. Mordant solution.

    Ferric ammonium sulfate (iron alum)
    (purple crystals only)   2.5 gm
    Distilled water   100 ml

2. 70% alcohol.

3. Hematoxylin solution.

    Hematoxylin crystals   10 gm
    Absolute alcohol   100 ml

    This solution should be well ripened for 2 to 3
    months.

4. Working solution.

    Ripened hematoxylin   5 ml
    Distilled water   100 ml

PROCEDURE

1. Wash blocks of tissue for 1 hour in running tap
    water.
2. Cut frozen sections at 20 to 30 microns into dis-
    tilled water.
3. Place sections in mordant solution for 6 hours.
4. Rinse in distilled water.
5. Place in 70% alcohol for 10 minutes.
6. Stain in hematoxylin solution for 10 to 24 hours.
7. Rinse in distilled water.
8. Differentiate in fresh 2.5% ferric ammonium sulfate,
    controlling under the microscope until the myelin
    stands out against a clear background; sections may
    be rinsed in distilled water during this procedure.
9. Wash thoroughly in distilled water, then place in
    tap water for 1 to 2 hours.
10. With the aid of a dissection needle or camel's hair
    brush, mount the sections on a slide and blot gently
    with fine filter paper.
11. From a dropper bottle dehydrate with 95% alcohol,
    then in absolute alcohol.
12. Pour on xylene from a dropper bottle until clear.
13. Mount in Permount.

Results. Myelin sheaths: blue-black.

Ref.   Mallory, F. B., Pathological Technique,
          Hafner Publishing Co., New York, 1961.

WEIL'S METHOD TO DEMONSTRATE MYELIN SHEATHS

Fixation. 10% formalin or Helly's fluid.

SOLUTIONS

1. Hematoxylin solution (10%).

    Hematoxylin crystals   10 gm
    Absolute alcohol   100 ml

    Allow to ripen for at least 6 months.

2. Working solution 1% hematoxylin

    Alcoholic hematoxylin   10 ml
    Distilled water   90 ml

3. Ferric ammonium sulfate (iron alum)
    (purple crystals only)   4 gm
    Distilled water   100 ml

4. Iron hematoxylin solution.

    Solution 2   50 ml
    Solution 3   50 ml

    DIFFERENTIATING Solutions

1. Ferric ammonium sulfate (iron alum)
    (purple crystanls only)   4 gm
    Distilled water   100 ml

2. Sodium borate (borax)   10 gm
    Potassium ferricyanide   12.5 gm
    Distilled water   100 ml

3. Ammonium hydroxide 28%   6 drops
    Distilled water   100 ml

PROCEDURE

1. Cut paraffin sections to 10 to 15 microns.
2. Deparaffinize and hydrate sections.
3. Remove mercury crystals.
4. Wash well in distilled water.
5. Stain for 30 minutes at 50°C in iron hematoxylin
    solution.
6. Wash in two changes of tap water.
7. Differentiate in 5% ferric ammonium sulfate until
    gray mater can just be distinguished.
8. Wash in three changes of tap water.

9. Continue differentiation in borax ferricyanide solution. Control differntiation under the micro-scope.
10. Wash in tap water, two changes.
11. Wash sections in dilute ammonia water.
12. Wash in distilled water.
13. Dehydrate in two changes of 95% alcohol, 5 minutes.
14. Clear in absolute alcohol, two changes, 5 minutes. each.
15. Clear in several changes of xylene.
16. Mount in Permount.

Results   Myelin sheaths: blue to blue-black.

Ref.   Weil, A.; Arch of Neurol and Phychiatry 26 1928 392-393

LOYEZ IRON HEMATOXYLIN METHOD TO DEMONSTRATE MYELIN

Fixation. 10% formalin.

SOLUTIONS

1.   Mordant solution.

     Ferric ammonium sulfate (iron alum)
     (purple crystals only)   4 gm
     Distilled water   100 ml

2.   Stock hematoxylin solution.

     Hematoxylin crystals   10 gm
     Absolute alcohol   100 ml

3.   Working solution: make up fresh each time.

     Stock hematoxylin solution   10 ml
     Distilled water   90 ml
     Saturated aqueous lithium carbonate   2 ml

4.   Weigert's differentiating fluid.

     Sodium borate (borax)   2 gm
     Potassium ferricyanide   2.5 gm
     Distilled water   200 ml

PROCEDURE

1.   Cut paraffin sections at 20 to 25 micorns.
2.   Deparaffinize and hydrate sections.

3. Mordant sections in iron alum for 24 hours.
4. Wash rapidly in tap water, two or three changes.
5. Place sections in hematoxylin solution at 37°C for 24 hours.
6. Wash in tap water for 5 to 10 minutes.
7. Differentiate in fresh 4% iron alum solution. As soon as the gray matter starts to clear and some detail can be seen in the white matter with the low power of the microscope, wash the sections well in tap water.
8. Differentiate further in Weigert's differentiator until myelin stands out.
9. Wash in tap water adding a few drops of 28% ammonium hydroxide per 100 ml if the water is not naturally alkaline.
10. Dehydrate in absolute alcohol, two changes.
11. Clear in two changes of xylene.
12. Mount in Permount.

Results.   Myelinated fibers: black, Gray matter: black. Red blood corpuscles, neuroglia, nuclei, and nucleoli of neurons: black.

Ref.   Loyez, M., C. R. Seanc. Soc. Biol., 69 (1910), 511

PAGE'S METHOD TO DEMONSTRATE MYELIN

Fixation. 10% formalin or Helly's fluid.

SOLUTIONS

1. Place 0.2 gm solochrome cyanin R.S. (C.I. No. 43820)* in a 250 ml flask and add 0.5 ml of concentrated sulfuric acid. Effervescence occurs, and a thick solution of creamy consistency is formed. Stir well to incorporate all the dye. Add 90 ml of distilled water and 10 ml of ferric ammonium sulfate (iron alum). Mix and filter. The solution keeps for months.

2. Differentiating solution.

    Ferric ammonium sulfate (iron alum)
    (purple crystals only)   10 gm
    Distilled water   100 ml

*Solochrome cyanin R.S., Robox Surgical Instrument, Co., Inc., Washington, D.C.

PROCEDURE

1. Deparaffinize and hydrate sections.
2. Remove mercury crystals if necessary.
3. Stain in solochrome solution for 10 minutes at room temperature.
4. Wash well in running tap water until blue.
5. Differentiate in 10% iron alum until nuclei are scarcely visible and muscle and connective tissue are colorless, about 10 to 15 minutes. Control under microscope.
6. Wash well in running tap water for 5 to 10 minutes. (Sections may be left in water for a few hours.)
7. Counterstain in dilute safranin or neutral red if desired.
8. Dehydrate in absolute alcohol.
9. Clear in xylene.
10. Mount in Permount.

Results.   Myelin: bright blue.   Other tissue elements: as counterstained.

Ref.   Page, K.M., J. Med. Tech., 22 (1965), 224-225.

VON BRAUNMUHL'S METHOD TO DEMONSTRATE SENILE PLAQUES

Fixation. 10% formalin

SOLUTIONS

1. Silver nitrate.

Silver nitrate	20 gm
Distilled water	100 ml

2. 28% ammonium hydroxide.

3. 40% formaldehyde.

4. Toning solution.

   1:500 aqueous yellow gold chloride.

5. Sodium hyposulfite solution.

Sodium hyposulfite	5 gm
Distilled water	100 ml

PROCEDURE

1. Cut frozen sections at 15 to 20 microns into distilled water.
2. Wash well in fresh distilled water.
3. Place sections in the silver nitrate solution in 50°C oven for 30 minutes to 1 hour. The sections should lie flat on the bottom of the dish and not overlap.
4. Remove sections from the oven and let cool slightly.
5. Prepare a row of three Petri dishes, the first containing 20 drops of 28% ammonium hydroxide in 80 ml of distilled water, the second distilled water, and the third 20 ml of 40% formaldehyde in 80 ml of distilled water.
6. Individaul sections are placed in the first dish (ammonium hydroxide) for 3 to 7 seconds; keep dish covered. Wash rapidly in distilled water. Place sections in third dish (formalin) for 2 to 3 seconds.
7. Wash tissue well in distilled water and examine under microscope. If fibers do not stand out, repeat cycle of ammonia, water, and formalin.
8. Tone in yellow gold chloride for 10 minutes.
9. Wash in distilled water.
10. Fix in sodium thiosulfate for 5 minutes.
11. Wash in distilled water.
12. Mount sections on slide and blot with fine filter paper.
13. From a dropper bottle pour on 95% alcohol, then absolute alcohol.
14. Clear in xylene in the same manner.
15. Mount in Permount.

Results. Senile plaques: black. Background: gray.

Ref.   Romeis, B., Mikroskopische Technik, 16th ed. Leibniz Verlag, Munich, 1968. 472.

PUTT'S METHOD TO DEMONSTRATE NISSL SUBSTANCE

Fixation. 10% formalin.

SOLUTIONS

1. Thionin solution. (Filter before use)

   To 10 ml of absolute alcohol add 1 ml of fresh aniline oil, shake well, make up to 100 ml with distilled water. To this add 0.25 gm of thionin.

2.   Differentiating solution.

Absolute alcohol   100 ml
Glacial acetic acid   2 to 3 drops

PROCEDURE

1.   Cut paraffin sections at 10 microns.
2.   Deparaffinize and hydrate sections.
3.   Rinse in distilled water.
4.   Stain in thionin solution for 5 minutes.
5.   Differentiate sections individually in acetic - alco-
     hol, controlling the degree under the microscope.
6.   Rinse quickly in absolute alcohol. This continues
     differentiation.
7.   Clear in xylene.
8.   Mount in Permount.

Results.   Nissl bodies and nucleoli of neurons; deep
            blue. The nuclear material and cytoplasm are
            pale blue or pink due to the polychrome nature
            of the dye. Nuclei of neuroglia cells; deep
            blue. Cytoplasm: pale blue.

Note.   The staining solution may be used repeatedly;
            filter before use.

Ref.   Putt, F. A., J. Neurosur., 2 (1948) 211.

PUTT'S METHOD TO DEMONSTRATE NISSLE SUBSTANCE ON OLD
FORMALIN-FIXED MATERIAL

Fixation. 10% formalin.

SOLUTIONS

1.   Thionin solution (filter before use). To 10 ml of
     absolute alcohol add 1 ml of fresh aniline oil,
     shake well, and make up to 100 ml with distilled
     water. To this add 0.25 gm of thionin.

2.   Differentiating solution (increasing the alcohol
     will speed up differentiation).

Aniline oil   25 ml
95% ethyl alcohol   25 ml

Gothard's differentiator (alternative solution, if
differentiation is too slow).

Pure creosote	50 ml
Cajeput oil	40 ml
Xylene	50 ml
Absolute alcohol	150 ml

PROCEDURE

1. Embed tissue in paraffin or celloidin.
2. Hydrate paraffin sections.
3. Stain sections in thionin solution overnight. As an alternative the sections may be placed in the staining solution, which is then heated to steaming and allowed to cool. The sections are removed after 15 minutes. Celloidin sections should be placed in a porcelain dish and heated over an alcohol flame.
4. Differentiate in aniline - alcohol or Gothard solution until the Nissl substance stands out; control under microscope.
5. Clear in Cajeput-xylene mixture for 5 to 15 minutes. Gothard's solution in absolute alcohol.
6. Rinse well in xylene.
7. Mount in Permount.

Results.   Nissl bodies and nuclei: deep blue. Nucleoli: purplish blue. Cytoplasm: pale blue.

Ref.   Gothard, C. R., Soc. Biol., 5 (1898). Putt, F. A., Unpublished.

EINARSONS'S GALLOCYANIN METHOD TO DEMONSTRATE NISSL SUBSTANCE

Fixation. 95% alcohol, 10% formalin, Helly's or Zenker's fluids.

SOLUTIONS.

1. 1 gm chromalum (chromium potassium sulfate) is dissolved in 200 ml of distilled water to which is added 0.3 gm of gallocyanin. The mixture is then gradually warmed and gently boiled for 15 to 30 minutes, shaking frequently. Cool gradually and then filter.

PROCEDURE

1. Embed tissue in paraffin.
2. Cut sections at 8 to 10 microns.
3. Deparaffinize and hydrate sections.
4. Remove mercury crystals if necessary.

5. Wash in distilled water
6. Stain in gallocyanin solution progressively 24
   to 48 hours or 3 to 4 hours at 50 C. When fresh,
   the solution stains more rapidly.
7. Wash in distilled water.
8. **Dehydrate** in 95% alcohol.
9. Dehydrate in absolute alcohol.
10. Clear in xylene.
11. Mount in Permount.

Results. Nissl substance: blue-black.

Ref.   Einarson, L. Amer. J. Path., 8 (1932), 295-309.

EINARSON'S GALLAMINE BLUE METHOD TO DEMONSTRATE NISSL
SUBSTANCE

Fixation. 95% alcohol, 10% formalin, Helly's or Zenker's
          fluids.

SOLUTIONS

1. Gradually heat 5/10 gm of gallamine blue in 200 ml
   of distilled water and allow to boil gently for 5 to
   10 minutes. Cool slowly and filter.
2. 50% and **70%** and **80%** alcohol.

PROCEDURE

1. Embed tissue in paraffin.
2. Cut sections at 8 to 10 microns.
3. Deparaffinize and hydrate sections.
4. Remove mercury crystals if necessary.
5. Wash in distilled water.
6. Stain in gallamine blue solution overnight.
7. Wash in distilled water for 5 to 10 minutes.
8. Differentiate in 50% alcohol for 15 seconds to 2
   minutes. Control under microscope.
9. Place sections in 70%, 80%, and 95%, and absolute
   alcohol for 3 minutes each. The dye is removed in
   the lower grades of alcohol, less in the higher.
10. Clear in two changes of xylene.
11. Mount in Permount.

Results. Nissl substance: blue-black.

Ref.   Einarson, L. Amer. J. Path., 8 (1932), 295-
           309.

RANVIER'S METHOD TO DEMONSTRATE MOTOR END PLATES

<u>Fixation</u>. Cut muscle in 3 to 5 mm slices and place in
fresh-filtered lemon juice for 10 to 15
minutes or 20% formic acid for the same time.
Handle tissue with paraffin coated forceps.

PROCEDURE

1. Pour off lemon juice and add 1% aqueous brown gold
    chloride in volume at least 10:1 of tissue; let
    stand for 10 to 60 minutes. (Formic acid material
    is rinsed in distilled water and stained for 20
    minutes in gold chloride, then rinsed in distilled
    water.
2. Transfer directly to 25% aqueous formic acid and
    reduce in the dark for 8 to 12 hours. (After rinsing,
    formic acid material is placed in 20% aqueous
    formic acid for 1 day in the dark.)
3. Wash in distilled water and place in a 50:50 mixture
    of glycerin and 50% alcohol; tissues may be left
    in this mixture for months until ready for mounting.
4. With dissecting needles tease out small fragments of
    tissue and place them on a 3 x 1 microslide in a
    small drop of pure glycerin; cover with a 22-mm
    cover slip and gently press down with a dissecting
    needle so that the preparation is a single-fiber
    thick; examine under microscope. If sections are
    satisfactory, they can be sealed with Permount.

<u>Results</u>.   Nerve fibers and endings: black. Other tissue
elements: various shades of purple or violet.

<u>Ref.</u>   Ranvier, J. L.; Quart. J. Microscop. Sci.,
<u>20</u> (1880), 465-458.

A BENZIDINE METHOD TO DEMONSTRATE THE VASCULAR PATTERN
OF THE CENTRAL NERVOUS SYSTEM

<u>Fixation</u>. 10% formalin for 1 to 2 weeks. Do not perfuse.

SOLUTIONS

1. Dissolve 0.5 gm of benzidine in 50 ml of absolute
    alcohol. Dissolve 0.1 gm of sodium nitroprusside in
    10 ml of distilled water. Mix the two solutions and
    make up to 100 ml with distilled water.

2. Absolute alcohol   50 ml
    Glacial acetic acid   2 ml
    30% hydrogen peroxide   0.5 ml
    Sodium nitroprusside   0.8 gm
    Distilled water   100 ml

    Dissolve the sodium nitroprusside in part of the
    distilled water, then bring the volume up to 100 ml.

PROCEDURE

1.   Wash tissue blocks in running tap water for 1 hour.
2.   Cut frozen sections at 200 to 300 microns into dis-
     tilled water.
3.   Wash well in distilled water for 30 minutes.
4.   Stain in the benzidine solution for 10 minutes.
5.   Wash rapidly in distilled water for 10 seconds.
6.   Stain in solution 2 until the vascular pattern
     stands out against a light background, placing the
     solution in $37^{o}C$ oven if necessary.
7.   Wash in distilled water.
8.   Dehydrate in **70% alcohol**, then in 95% alcohol, each
     acidulated with 2% glacial acetic acid.
9.   Dehydrate in absolute alcohol, two changes.
10. Clear in xylene.
11. Mount on slides and coverslip in Permount.

Results.   Vascular pattern stands out blue against a
           colorless background.

Ref.   Doherty, M. M., Suh, T. H. and Alexander,
           L.; Arch. Neurol. **Psychiate.**, 40 (1938), 158-162,
           Copyright 1938, American Medical Association.

Note.   The finsihed preparation should be kept away
           from light and heat or fading will occur.

A **Method of Staining Macroscopic Brain Sections**

Fixation. 10% formalin.

SOLUTIONS

1.   Mulligan's phenol solution.

     Phenol crystals (melted   4 ml
     Cupric sulfate, ($CuSO4$ $5H2O$) **Crystals**   0.5 gm
     Concentrated hydrochloric acid   0.125 ml
     Distilled water   100 ml

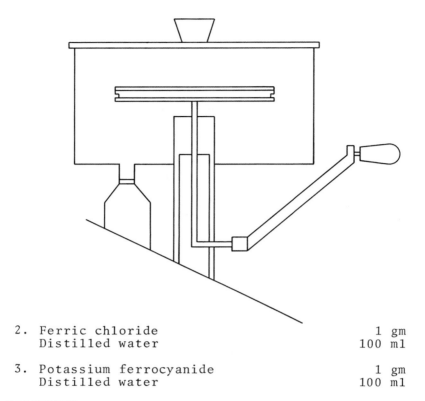

2. Ferric chloride   1 gm
   Distilled water   100 ml

3. Potassium ferrocyanide   1 gm
   Distilled water   100 ml

PROCEDURE

1. Cut thin slices of a well-fixed brain to the desired
   thickness with a brain knife coated with glycerin.
2. Wash in running tap water for 12 to 24 hours.
3. Wash in distilled water for 1 hour, change water
   three or four times.
4. Place sections in Mulligan's phenol solution preheated to 60°C for 2 minutes.
5. Rinse sections in a large volume of cold tap water
   for 1 minute.
6. Place in ferric chloride solution for 2 minutes.
7. Wash in running tap water for 5 minutes.
8. Place in ferrocyanide solution until gray matter is
   brilliant blue. (Approximately 3 minutes, no longer.)
9. Wash overnight in running tap water.
10. Preserve in 70% alcohol.

Ref. LeMasurier, J. E., Arch. Neur. Psychiat., 34
     (1935), 1065, Mulligan, J. H., J. Anat., 65
     (1931), 468-472.

Chapter 13

GROSS SPECIMEN PRESERVATION FOR TEACHING PURPOSES

Brady 1

Potassium sulfate	6 gm
Potassium nitrate	114 gm
Sodium chloride	54 gm
Sodium bichromate	60 gm
Sodium sulfate	66 gm
Chloral hydrate	300 gm
Formaldehyde 40%	300 ml
Distilled water	10,000 ml

Dissolve the solids in the distilled water, then add the formaldehyde.

PROCEDURE

1. Cut section and trim off all excess tissue before fixation.
2. Place specimen in jar or vat with cotton around it to prevent contact with bottom or sides of jar.
3. Adequate fixation depends on the size of the speciman 3 to 10 days will be sufficient for all specimens.
4. Usually specimens fixed in Brady are not used for histological purposes, but if this should be necessary, place selected tissue directly into 10% formalin.

PALKOWSKI METHOD TO PRESERVE GROSS SPECIMENS IN A PLIABLE CONDITION

Fixation. Modified Kaiserling's solution (Brady No. 1).

SOLUTION

Chloral hydrate	300 gm
Potassium sulfate	6 gm
Potassium nitrate	114 gm

311

Sodium chloride   54 gm
Sodium sulfate   66 gm
Sodium bicarbonate   60 gm
Formaldehyde 40%   300 ml
Distilled water   10,000 ml

Dissolve the solids in the distilled water, then add the formaldehyde.

PROCEDURE

1. Fix specimen as soon as possible for 3 to 4 hours in four times its volume of modified Kaiserling's solution. Solid organs should not exceed 3 cm in thickness; cut lungs in half along planes of major bronchi and submerge under cotton staurated with fixative.
2. Drain away excess fixative and place specimen in four times its volume of 80% alcohol for 18 to 24 hours.
3. Place specimen in polyethlene bag not much larger. than specimen, seal, and freeze at -20°F. Specimens keep indefinitely and retain their original color, become pliable after thawing, and can be returned to the deep freeze with only little deterioration for subsequent use.

Ref.   Palkowski, W., Tech. Bull. Reg. Med. Tech., 30 (1960), 493.

Chapter 14

MODIFIED GOUGH AND WENTWORTH METHOD
TO MOUNT WHOLE ORGANS ON PAPER

Fixation. Whole lungs may be perfused with 10% formalin or 3 1/2% glutaraldehyde according to the method described by Heard or Gough and Wentworth. Slice fixed lung into sagittal sections about 3/4 in. thick. One-inch sections of other organs may be fixed for about 1 week in 10% formalin (glutaraldehyde is less suitable as the rate of penetration is too slow). Wash the sections in running tap water for 2 days to remove all traces of formalin. A small gauze bag of thymol added to the wash will prevent the growth of fungi. The balance of the procedure should be carried out in a formalin-free, preferably air-conditioned, room.

PROCEDURE

1. Infiltrate and embed sections in the following solution:

Gelatin (100 bloom, Kind and Knox)	600 gm
Cellosolve (ethylene glycol monoethyl ether)	120 ml
Clycerin	300 ml
Caprylic alcohol	15 ml
Warm water	3750 ml
Thymol	pinch

    Dissolve with the aid of heat on a water bath; gentle agitation with an electric stirrer will spped up solution.
2. Place the sections in hot (60°C) gelatin solution in a suitable container deep enough to allow the specimen to be fully submerged. (Aluminum Teflon lined baking pans are useful.)

3. Place the container in a vacuum oven regulated to 24 to 30 mm of Hg 1/2 hour to infiltrate and remove trapped air. This step is necessary for lungs only. Omit step 3 when handling solid organs such as liver or kidneys.

4. Transfer the container to a 37°C oven for 24 hours; specimen should remain flat. Covering the container (Saran wrap is handy) reduces loss of water from evaporation.

5. Place the container in refrigerator to solidify the gelatin. When the gelatin is solid, gently heat the pan in warm water and invert to remove the block. Trim off excess gelatin from sides, leaving blocks square or rectangular. These blocks may be wrapped in Saran and kept in the refrigerator until ready for mounting.

6. Heat the specimen holder in hot water. Then, **supporting** the plate on a flat surface, place the gelatin block on the warm plate; this melts the undersurface. Cool the plate over cold water to reset the gelatin; the block will adhere to the plate. Place in a deep-freeze cabinet at -25°C for 3 to 4 hours depending on the size and thickness of the block. Specimens may be left overnight or longer if necessary.

7. Section on large MSE microtome. Prolonged freezing leaves the gelatin too hard to section, but it may be softened by applying a cloth dampened with hot water. When the gelatin has reached the proper temperature, sectioning may proceed without interruption. We usually cut sections at 300 microns depending on the consistency of the tissue.

8. Receive cut sections into the following solution:

Formaldehyde 40%	500 ml
Sodium acetate	200 gm
Water	5000 ml

Leave sections in solution for 24 to 48 hours to harden the gelatin, sections may be left immersed for longer periods of time without harm. Wash in running tap water for 1 to 2 hours to remove all traces of formalin. Sections to be stained are placed directly into hot water for at least 3 to 4 changes or until all traces of gelatin have been removed. These sections may be stained immediately or transfered to 10% formalin in a covered dish for storage. Formalin should be removed from stored sections by washing a few minutes in running tap water just prior to staining.

9. Mounting gelatin; No. 225.

    Gelatin   450 gm
    Glycerin   280 ml
    Cellosolve   160 ml
    Hot water   3400 ml

    Dissolve as outlined for embedding gelatin. Keep solu-
    tion warm during use. Place a 10 x 12-in. piece of
    Plexiglass (glass cannot be used, since the section
    will not strip off) on a flat surface on some type of
    support with facilities to catch the excess gelatin.
    Pour a little warm gelatin over the entire surface of
    the plate and orient the section, removing the excess
    embedding gelatin from around the edges and from the
    plate. Make certain that the section is flat and free
    from folds. Add more gelatin and cover the section
    with a 10 x 12-in. sheet of Whatman's No. 1 filter
    paper. Gently roll a rubber squeegee over the paper
    (Kodak, 12-in. type) to remove excess gelatin and air
    bubbles. Stand the Plexiglass sheet (with section at-
    tached) on end for a few minutes to drain. Place the
    plate in an x-ray drier overnight or dry at room tem-
    perature. When thoroughly dry, gently strip the paper
    with section attached from the Plexiglass. Trim away
    excess paper and lightly coat specimen side with
    Krylon clear spray. (This prevents the films from
    sticking together in humid weather.)

    We have found that specimens containing excessive
    blood have a tendency to stick to Plexiglass. This can
    be overcome by mounting such tissue on thin Mylar film
    in the same manner as described above. These thin
    films can be supported during mounting on a piece of
    Plexiglass, removed, and dried flat at room tempera-
    ture. The drying time is more rapid than for Plexi-
    glass-mounted sections.

    If suitable, the balance of the uncut tissue may be
    washed free of gelatin in hot water and sealed in
    polyethylene bags containing a little formalin. These
    specimens are useful for gross demonstration.

10. Staining. To stain this type of tissue, all dyes must
    be greatly diluted. We have used Bullard's hematoxylin
    counterstained with Lendrum's phloxine-calcium
    chloride, Van Gieson for connective tissue, Alcian
    blue for mucin, and iron stains. Other methods are
    in the process of development and will be published
    when acceptable results are attained.

11. Mounting stained sections. Straighten out a section
     on the bottom of a dish of shallow water, gently
     press a rectangular piece of filter paper over the
     section until contact is made. Holding the tip of the
     section in place against the paper, slowly withdraw
     one end of the paper at an angle; the section will
     adhere and follow the paper. Place the paper with
     the section side down onto a piece of Plexiglass
     covered with warm gelatin mounting solution, gently
     peel away the paper, and straighten out the section.
     Carefully, wipe away any excess gelatin from
     around the section. Allow the plate to dry over-
     night on a flat surface.

     Transfer the section to paper by pouring warm mount-
     ing gelatin solution over the plate and rolling
     as outlined above. Allow to dry overnight. When
     thoroughly dry, strip off the film and spray with
     Krylon.

12. Saran wrap mounting. Sections mounted on paper are
     subject to compression. To overcome this condition
     in tissues to be examined in depth with the dissect-
     ing microscope, place the tissues as they are section-
     ed directly into glycerin and allow to clear for 24
     hours. Place in fresh glycerin for an additional
     24 to 48 hours depending on the number to be cleared.
     (If serial sections are desired, place a numbered
     piece of onionskin paper between each section;
     this procedure is best carried out by two people.)
     Occasional gentle agitation will facilitate proper
     cleaning. When the sections are cleared, place the
     individual tissues on a piece of Saran Wrap about
     twice the size of the section, gently blot away any
     excess glycerin, leaving enough to keep the section
     moist. Double the Saran Wrap over the section and
     fold in all the edges to form an envelope. These
     sections keep indefinitely without evaporation.
     Stained and unstained tissues and specimens injected
     with various colored gelatins to demonstrate vascular
     patterns may be preserved in this manner.

Ref.   Heard, B. E., Thorax, 13 (1958).
              Gough J. and Wentworth, J. E. Personal Commun-
              ication.
              Carrington, C. B., Putt, F. A. and Powell, A.;
              Modified Gough and Wentworth Method, unpublished
              Hales, M. R. and Carrington, C. B.; A pigmented

gelatin mass for vascular injection, Yale J. Biol.
Med., 43 (1971), 257-270.

Equipment and Supplies to Process Gough Sections

1   12 cu. ft. refrigerator and freezer - must be frost
     free (domestic type).

1   Thelco Incubator Model 6, Cat. No. L-17011, Will
     Scientific Inc.

1   Paper cutter, 15 x 16 1/2 "Popular," Milton Bradley
     Co., Springfield, Mass.

1   Kodak paper roller, 12-in. size.

1   Vacuum pump, Fisher Scientific Co., New York.

2   dozen Plexiglass sheets, 10 x 12 in.

1   Dish - rack for rolling out prints (homemade).

1   Roll clear acetate film, 40 in. wide x 100 ft long,
     0.010 in. thickness, Ridout Plastics, San Diego,
     Calif.

50 lb Gelatin, 100 Bloom LINE bone gelatin, Kind and Knox
     Gelatin Co., Camden, N. J.

Saran Wrap, 12-in. size, 2000 ft, Harlem Paper Products
Bronx, N. Y.

Glycerine.
Ethylene glycol.
Caprylic alcohol.
Thymol.
Sodium acetate, Fisher Scientific Co.,

100 sheets, Whatman No. 1 Filter Paper 46 x 57 cm. Fisher
     Scientific Co.

Krylon Spray (clear), Fisher Scientific Co., New York.

1   MSE large section microtome, (Gough and Wentworth)
     with 9 x 11 in. table including knife clamps.

1   MSE microtome knife, 350-mm long, wedge shaped.

1   knife handle.

1   Knife back, Instrumentation Associates, Inc., New York.

1   Revco Sub-Zero cabinet Model No. RSZ 503, 5 cu. ft.
     Capacity, temperature to -50°F, Revco Inc. Deerfield,
     Mich.

1   National Vacuum Oven, Cat. No. 13-262-12 V3,
     Fisher Scientific Co.

Chapter 15

WEIBEL'S METHOD TO MOUNT SECTIONS IN PLASTIC FILM

The use of plastic as a medium for mounting stained sections in film form is a convenient method for preparing and storing routine or serial sections in compact form.

<u>Fixation</u>. Any routine fixative.

<u>Method</u>.   Paraffin.

<u>Equipment</u>.

1.   A modified hand-driven centrifuge as illustrated, with rotating table, clips, and receptacle for excess paraffin.

2.   Glass staining dishes: Fisher Scientific Co., No. 15-240.

3.   Plastic: Cyclon-Lack Farblos No. 10830, lufttrock- nend.*

4.   Thinner: Cyclon-Lack Verduennung L.[†]

PROCEDURE

1.   Clean glass plates thoroughly.   Number plate with diamond pencil; this will transfer to film when stripped from glass plate.
2.   Cut paraffin sections at 5 microns and mount sections of ribbon in proper order on an albuminized glass plate.   (A tissue flotation bath may be used but the slide warming table method is more convenient.)
3.   Drain excess water from slide and place in 37°C oven overnight to dry.
4.   Deparaffinize and stain as desired in large glass trays.

*Naegely, Eschmann & Cie.   AG, Lack- und Farbenfabrik, Zurich, Switzerland.

5. Dehydrate through alcohols to xylene, then place in
    a mixture of absolute alcohol and xylene in equal
    parts.
6. Place slide on table of centrifuge and clip in
    place; allow excess fluid to remain on slide
7. Pour ample plastic onto the center of the plate.
    Cover the centrifuge immediately and spin gently,
    gradually increasing speed for a few turns. The
    intensity of spinning is a matter of experience,
    depending on the consistency of the plastic, and
    the desired thickness of the film. (Films that are
    too thick are generally better than films that are
    too thin, since these have a tendency to wrinkle.)
8. Dry for 24 hours in a well-ventilated, dust free
    room. If many sections are to be processed, a hood
    is recommended, since the fumes contain toxic
    organic solvents.
9. Incise edges of films by scratching along the edges
    of the glass plate with the back of an old knife
    or razor blade. Soak in cold or lukewarm water for
    2 hours. Peel off films gently and dry between fil-
    ter paper. Mark films with pen and India ink.

Storage of Films. Place films between sheets of tracing
paper, which are stapled together on one side to form a
booklet. If films have a tendency to wrinkle, press
these booklets overnight in a large book. The booklets
may be bound in a cardboard or minila folder and then
labeled.

Microscopy. For microscopy, the film is placed on a
large glass slide. Good optical quality and minimal
thickness are required for good results. If wrinkled,
flatten film with soft brush. For visual observation,
regular dry system objectives with initial magnification
of 20X can be used. Oil immersion can be used directly
on the films; for optimal results, a drop of oil should
also be placed underneath the section.

Secondary Mounting in Permount. Single sections can be
mounted in Permount. Individual sections are cut out
with scissors and placed on a drop of Permount on a
slide. A second drop is placed on the film and a coverslip applied. If large sections are mounted, small lead
weights should be placed on the coverslip overnight.

Ref.   Weible, E., personal communication; Department
        of Pathology, YALE University School of Med-
        icine.

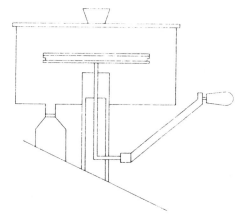

BIBLIOGRAPHY

Baker, J. R., Cytological Technique, 3rd ed., John Wiley and Sons, Inc., New York, 1950.

Baker, J. R., Principles of Biological Microtechnique, John Wiley and Sons, Inc., New York 1958.

Carlton, H. M. and Drury, R. A. B., Histological Technique, 3rd ed., Oxford University Press, 1957.

Conn, H. J., Biological Stains, Lillie, R. D. (ed.) 8th ed., Biotech Publications, Geneva, N. Y. 1969.

Davenport, H. A., Histological and Histochemical Technics, W. B. Saunders Co., Philadelphia, 1960.

Emmel, V. M. and Cowdry, E. V., Laboratory Technique in Biology and Medicine, 4th ed., The Williams and Wilkins Co., Baltimore, 1964

Gray, Peter, The Microtomist's Formulary and Guide Constable and Co. Ltd., London, 1954.

Gray, Peter, Handbook of Basic Microtechnique, McGraw-Hill Book Co., New York, 1952.

Gridley, M. F., Manual of Histologic and Special Staining Technics, 2nd ed., McGraw-Hill Book Co., New York, 1960.

Gurr, Edward, Encyclopedia of Microscopic Stains, The Williams and Wilkins Co., Baltimore, 1960.

Gurr, Edward, Staining, Practical and Theoretical, The Williams and Wilkins Co., Baltimore, 1962.

Humason, G. L., Animal Tissue Techniques, W. H. Freeman and Co., San Francisco, 1962.

Jones, Ruth McClung, McClung's Handbook of Microscopical Techniques, Paul B. Hoeber, Inc., Harper and Row, New York, 1950.

Lee, A. B., in J. B. Gatenby and T. S. Painter (eds)
    The Microtomist's Vade-Mecum, 10th ed., McGraw-Hill
    Book Co., New York, 1937.

Lillie, R. D., Histopathologic Technic and Practical
    Histochemistry, 3rd ed., McGraw-Hill Book Co.
    New York, 1965.

Liggett, W. F., Ancient and Medieval Dyes, Chemical
    Publishing Co., Inc., Brooklyn, New York, 1944.

Mallory, F. B., Pathological Technique, Hafner Publishing
    Co., Inc., New York, 1968.

McManus, J. F. A., and Mowry, R.W., Staining Methods;
    Histologic and Histochemical, Harper and Row, Hoeber
    Medical Division, New York, 1960.

Pearse, A. G. E., Histochemistry, Theoretical and Applied
    Little, Brown and Co., Boston, 1960.

Steedman. H. A., Section Cutting in Microscopy, Blackwell
    Scientific Publications, Oxford, 1960.

INDEX